The

Food Life

Written by Travis Woo

Edited By Vincent Ferraiuolo & Alexander Hinkley

Art by Sean MacClain

Cover by Pia Pulido

The Food Life

Coming Home

Food Lifestyle

Food Lives

Food Society

Poems and Reads

Coming Home

In Pursuit of Good Food

Like you, I get hungry. And when I'm hungry I want to eat. And when I eat, I want to eat good food. That's all. I started by following my taste and hunger, but while eating junk food lit up my brain with pleasure, I didn't feel my best after. I watched "Supersize Me" and felt as sick as the protagonist eating McDonald's three meals a day. I wanted to eat good, but I wanted to feel good too. I began to follow my gut which led me to organic restaurants, health food stores, and farmer's markets. This food was also delicious, and I felt even better after I ate it. Looking at the food in front of me I started to wonder - where did this come from?

I read Michael Pollan's "Omnivore's Dilemma" and was grossed out by how absurd the conventional food system is. I tried to wrap my head around the labyrinth flow of pesticided, herbicided, and fertilized grain, and the hundred million caged animals living on slats over manure lagoons who never step outside or have room to even turn around. The plants are bred for cardboard-like shelf stability for long-distance transportation over taste and nutrition. The animals are bred to put on the most

1

weight the fastest and are shot full of hormones and antibiotics to keep them alive just long enough for slaughter. I was disgusted and felt deceived. This was the food I had been eating all along? This is the system I had been paying my money towards? I took the red pill. Now that I knew, I couldn't keep on eating how I had been eating. Wendell Berry once said, "To be interested in food but not food production is clearly absurd". So I decided to go deeper in my pursuit of good food. I sought out the source- the land where it was growing.

I walked by the local community garden and noticed a posting about Wednesday volunteer hours on the bulletin board. I came back to dig my hands in the soil and breath in the sweet earthy aroma. I brought my kitchen scraps to feed the garden. I turned the compost. I picked the brains of the other volunteers. I left with fresh kale, chard, garlic, onions, berries and an invitation to volunteer on Friday at the local city farm. I arrived to weed strawberries, feed goats, harvest potatoes, broccoli, collards, and chard, to plant leeks, garlic, and purples onions. I left with a backpack full of produce and came back for solstice and fall celebrations. It was my first taste of The Food Life.

When the growing season ended for the winter I was sad and bored, so I flew South where the food grows year-round. My search led me to an organic, biodynamic farm producing food for the local communities I harvested their salad greens, carrots, beets, turnips, purplette onions, papayas, and mangos. I spread manure and mulch, prepared fields, transplanted baby brassicas, planted fruit trees, cared for the sheep, chickens, and pigs. In exchange, they fed me.

This was truly good food. It was organic. It was close to home. The soil was cared for. It was loved. The animals were happy. This food might wilt after a week on the shelf, but it didn't matter because it travelled just three feet from my knees to my mouth. It looked beautiful. It tasted great and I felt my best after. It filled me all the way up. There was no mystery where it came from. We did it as a team and we ate it together.

This is what I've learned about good food- it comes from healthy soil, happy plants, happy animals, and happy people. It comes from respect and love for nature. It comes from composting and recycling. It takes serious labor. It comes from nearby. It comes from hard working people coming together over a shared mission.

Good food may or may not be all around you. Food deserts in the middle of cities are unfortunately real. But the potential for good food is everywhere. Across the world, the soil is coming back to life. Community gardens are springing up alongside small box gardens, rooftop gardens, patio gardens, school gardens, and backyard hen houses. Young people like you and me are becoming disenchanted with modern lifestyle and going back to the land in search of good food. Older workers who have lost their jobs to automation are searching for something to do. The ancient lifestyle is still here, available to any of us who want it badly enough. Like many others, I've found deep in my bones The Food Life to be right for me, and it may be right for you too.

A Brief History of Food

There was probably a Big Bang. At one point everything was all crammed together, followed by a massive outward explosion of cosmic dust. Boom! Everything separated and expanded. From the swirling cosmic debris came stars, planets, moons, and the Earth.

Life was born in the seas. At first single cell organisms emerged from the primordial soup. Then multicellular organisms began to eat the single cell organisms. Then came more advanced life which split off into plants, fungi, and animals. Everything was eating everything else. Some of the animals moved from the seas to the supercontinent Pangaea. And then dinosaurs arrived (who somehow later evolved into modern chicken nuggets).

Then came humans, two million years ago, who walked on 2 legs, gathered, scavenged, and hunted small prey. About 300,000 years ago humans harnessed fire, allowing them to expand their dietary range and reduce their time chewing, giving them more energy to craft tools, sharpen hunting strategies, and grow larger brains. These ancient people lived in a different world. There was an abundance of giant, meaty land mammals, like the mastodon. There were lots of fruit and berries to collect. There weren't too many people, and the eating was good. But over time the biggest animals were hunted to extinction as the human population surged. The scale finally tipped.

About 10,000 years ago, people started keeping animals in herds and planting gardens in their communities. These plants and animals were domesticated by weeding out bad behavior and selecting and protecting good traits. In this way, our grazing herds became more docile and affectionate and our wild plants became sweeter and more nutritious. Farming was born.

Farming began independently in a few places-Middle Easterners domesticated wheat, goats, peas, and lentils; Chinese domesticated pigs, rice, and millet; South Americans domesticated llamas and potatoes; North Americans domesticated corn, beans, and pumpkins; Africans domesticated African millet, African rice, sorghum, and honey bees; New Guineans domesticated banana and sugar cane. Wherever farming didn't start independently it quickly spread, although a few remote areas where the wild eating was still good held out for a long time.

The switch from hunting and gathering to farming was not a direct step into garden paradise.

Humans gave up a lot. They traded in varied diets and freedom of movement for monotonous diets, arthritis, increased child mortality, diminished physical size, worse teeth, more disease, and longer work days. The new farm life wasn't all bad though. People were still working with plants and animals, but now they were cocreating directly with the Earth, deepening their relationship with God and nature. With grain stores and herds came increased food yield, increased food security, and greater confidence in the future. Populations exploded, and for better or worse, once farming started there was no going back to the old ways. Whether from choice or necessity, farming was the future.

With farming came food stockpiling and a percentage of the population was freed from having to work on food. Some people specialized on developing written language. Others could become professional soldiers, architects, artists, or priests. Civilization was born. Currency came as an exchange between farmers and various service workers. Roads, pack beasts, and wheels made better food transport and distribution, allowed the separation of farmland and living space, and more people began to congregate in cities

Farming civilizations spread across the world, from east to west until the good land ran out. Once all the land was claimed, efficiency became more important. So came the industrial revolution- farm machines and systemization allowed for more food yield with less labor, freeing even more people from farm work, who moved to the cities to work in factories with machines. Many of these factories made war machines, and then chemical fertilizers after the World Wars. Soldiers traded their guns for factory jobs, then chairs and desks of the tech revolution.

With the advent of steam ships, railroads, and planes, it became very easy to ship goods, such as seeds, fruits, and plant clippings. Government agent food explorers and plant entrepreneurs sought out and distributed the best varieties of crops from around the world. Everyone was treated to new and better foods. When previously people had only access to a few staple crops in their locale, they could know munch on tropical fruits and vegetables during their lunch breaks.

The advance of industry and technology greatly increased the possible output of food production. Huge machines, computer systems, and transportation networks allowed for massive food production with only a few people managing the systems and machinery. Within a short time, the backyard produce production dropped from 50% to almost nothing as the human population surged from millions to billions.

With increased quantity has come decreased quality, by necessity. It's difficult to feed billions of people. Thus, the birth of concentrated animal feeding operations, herbicide resistant crops, genetic modification of life. Thus, the abandonment of our most delicious 10,000-year-old heirlooms in favor of a few bland breeds prized for transport friendly shelf stability and herbicide resistance. Thus, the replacement of food with processed "food" products. In this new world, we have plenty of calories to support everyone, but perhaps not the vitamins, minerals, and nutrients to support good health.

Look at how far we've strayed from our ancestors. For millions of years we've participated with nature to gather and grow our food. But for the most recent 100 years- a tiny blip of time- we've been inside eating meat that is grown inside. No wonder so many people are unhappy, unhealthy, and turning to drugs and suicide. Disease, mental illness, and hysterics rule. Modern lifestyles and diets are extremely unnatural to our inner animal and our people are suffering.

There are some perks to the modern food landscape. It's never before been possible to eat as varied and healthy a diet irrespective of location and season. You can eat Mexican mangos, Alaskan salmon, and California greens almost anywhere in any one day of the year. It's never before been possible to farm as wide a variety of crops. You can order seeds online from anywhere in the world and they will arrive for you to plant within a week. While the lows are low, the highs are extremely high.

I'm optimistic about our food future. While farming isn't a perfect profession, more people are recognizing it as a return to normalcy and superior to the craziness of the modern world. As automation increases, more people will be freed from their jobs and they will be welcome in intensive farming. Organic farming and gardening might not scale as easily, but it makes more and better food with less land. Weeding 10,000 acres by hand may be lot more labor intensive than one person programming a machine to spray herbicide, but it produces more food, better food, and fewer sick people. We may be headed back that way.

I see one possible future with more community gardens, backyard gardens, school gardens, rooftop gardens, care gardens, and small farms with egg-laying hens in the city. A vibrant local food system supplying half the world's food. A reemphasis on taste and nutrition. Happier people, healthier people, alongside happier and healthier plants and animals.

I see another possible future with even more unnatural farming practices, tumor meat grown in labs, more chemical solutions, more waste. More unhealthy people, sick from an unnatural food system, overfed but under-nourished, left without the energy to get up and make a change for their lives, turning to more drugs and immersive virtual reality for a better life experience. Given the situation, it's hard to fault someone for plugging an IV into their vein and plugging their brain into the Matrix.

Einstein said we can't fix the problems of the 20th century with the same thinking that created them. Well, we have a whole new century of problems now, and while we need to look to the future for solutions, we should also look to our ancient heritage as agriculturists. Together we can make a better food system that goes beyond merely fulfilling our caloric needs, and prioritizes quality of life for plants, animals, humans, and the soil of Earth. We will return to The Food Life.

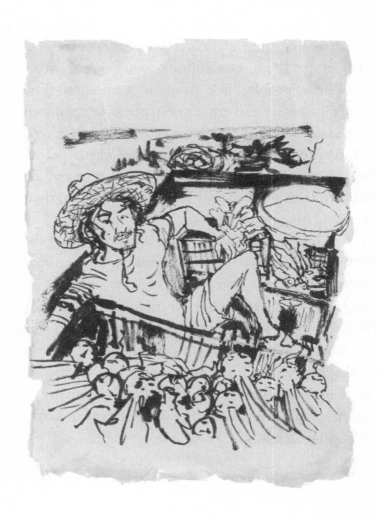

Around the World and Back to the Earth

I finally knew that this is what I needed to be doing with my life. The smells, sights, sensations, and sounds were familiar to me- a few glimpses from my youth, but more so flashbacks to past lives. Ancient memories came flooding back. I had been doing this for ten thousand years. It was thick in my blood. Yet I had never considered this in my lifetime until now. I had never been exposed to it. It had never been suggested to me. It was new, but I knew immediately that it was right. I could do this for the rest of my life. I was certain. I was home.

At 25 years old I was lost and searching. I had set out and accomplished most of my teenage goals. I had traveled, competed, written, and shared, but it had brought me only fleeting satisfaction. To be honest, my life wasn't particularly good. My days were blah. I had been driven by a mission, but I was missing a richness of experience. I was missing a team. I was missing something I couldn't quite put my finger on until I came here.

As a child I had weeded my mother's garden and harvested a few strawberries in the summertime. I remember scraps from the kitchen to the worm bin in the back yard. We were lucky to have room to grow a few plants. But I had no awareness of career farming. I never met a farmer or heard any discussion of it. As a city kid I was distracted by the bright lights. I wanted to play sports. I wanted to produce music. I wanted to play games. I wanted to travel. I wanted to write. I wanted to build businesses. I wanted to use the internet and monetize my hobbies.

As a young teen I read Tim Ferriss' "*The 4-Hour Workweek*" and it sent me on a different path from my peers. I saw a future possibility of separating money from time and doing whatever I wanted. My parents encouraged me to blaze my path, so long as I was diligent. I worked hard in school and tried out a variety of jobs- sports camp coach, food prep, restaurant server, office grunt, social media for nonprofit, retail, event staff, game design, and marketing.

Like many young men I played games, but I was more serious about it than most. I started competing and winning Magic: The Gathering tournaments and traveling nationally. Magic is a competitive card game with a cult following, millions of players, and a huge market. It grew as I grew. I began to write, blog, YouTube, and live stream. I served an audience and earned a paycheck. I looked in the future and saw a bright possibility, so I stuck with it through college, and as I graduated it became my ticket to turn the 4-Hour Workweek into a reality. It wasn't the most lucrative thing, but I was paid for my content, not for my time, and I was freed to do what I wanted.

What would you do if you separated your money from your time? At first you would probably spend more time on your hobbies. I spent more time producing music. But mostly I worked out. I knew that building a healthy foundation now would pay off for me later. So I trained on the football field, in the weight room, on the basketball court, on the beach, and in the pool. I stretched, did yoga, farm carries, and self-massage. At night I streamed Magic Online and produced content. I scrounged and saved my money with the goal of traveling abroad.

After almost two years, it was finally time to set out. I had placed in the Top 8 of a big tournament in Oakland with my brother and we both won airfare to Spain. We went together, but after the competition he returned home while I continued on. With money saved up, money coming in, and no reason to be anywhere in particular, I decided to stay awhile. After the tournament I headed up to the North coast to stay with a friend who was playing on a competitive basketball team. I went to practices where the coaches and players spoke in Spanish and stayed for a season. I wasn't a professional athlete, but it crossed another goal off my bucket list. I didn't care for it to be a permanent lifestyle, and I started to wonder what would be next.

I extended my trip by leaving Spain for the Southwest coast of England, a beautiful spot in the world. I moved into a surf hostel and spent a lot of time in the ocean. We collected mussels from the rocks, ate fresh fish, and made fires on the beach. For the first time I spent more than a week out of the city and grew an appreciation for the quiet skies and visible stars.

After my tourist visas ran out I returned home to Seattle, but I couldn't just go back to the same old life. I knew it was time to move on, but I wasn't sure to what. I needed new goals. I decided to get out of the city and move somewhere remote, beautiful, and affordable. From a Twitter recommendation I took a train and craigslist ride south to Northern California, where I continued training, playing, and producing But I was becoming bored and dissatisfied. You'd think so much freedom would make life awesome, but it left some things missing, and I wasn't sure what. To have something to look forward to I decided to visit friends in the same Spain to England loop in the next year, which passed more seasons, but didn't satisfy or inspire me. I spent another cold winter in Spain and realized in England that the vacation lifestyle of my friends in the lodge was a boring escape from reality. I returned home again at 25, now with an idea of what I was missing.

I had too much freedom and I was missing commitments, obligations, and responsibility to real life communities. I was too separated from everyday working society and I was missing mentors. I was stretching too much for meaning in my work and I was missing purpose in something I truly believed in. I was moving weights around when I wanted to be building something with teammates. I was moving around too much and I was missing intimate connections and certainty. I was too absorbed in the future and I was missing good todays. I was spending too much time online and I was missing the land. Finally, I knew what I was missing, and I could go out and find it.

I was on my way to catch the bus into town for a dental checkup when I walked by the Arcata Community Garden, a small plot of land on the corner. I saw vegetables, fruit, and flowers in small beds. I saw a compost heap. I smelled the Earth. This is what I was looking for.

I started working with the land every week at the Bayside Park Farm. I liked that it was physical and outside. I liked working with community members. I liked the smells and sensations. Working on the land with my friends became the highlight of my week. I loved leaving with fresh food that I had helped grow. This work mattered. These people cared. This land was loved. I was sad when the growing season ended but happy to celebrate the change of seasons on the farm with my new farmily.

I considered committing to farming full time but wasn't yet ready because I had gotten even more deeply involved with competitive Magic. I had a coaching business to run. I had content to create. I had tournaments to attend. I had to travel.

I drew the right card at the right time and took off for competitions across America, Europe, and the Pacific. My main focus was the game, but when I could I took extra time to visit local farms where I was traveling.

When the tour took me to Hawaii, I decided I would stay a month to search for farms and explore the possibility of living there. I was drawn to the climate and the people. They had a year-long growing season. I asked around and found my way to Kahumana Organic Farm and Café where I was lucky to meet the right person who offered to host me. I stayed a week to volunteer in what was basically a food village. Here was a community that lived on the land, worked on the land, and ate on the land. They had a lot of food growing, room to expand, a young passionate team, a long history, and great community involvement in a gorgeous space surrounded by mountains and ocean. I loved the taste and wanted to come back. So after another series of tournaments I did, taking a season off my grind to work on the land for three months.

I paid money to work for free. I didn't apply. I booked a room in their retreat centers and started showing up to work shifts. Having become bored with hobbies, travel, and leisure, I decided I would work on something I thought was really important. I went out into the heat and shoveled rows while my teammates rolled out irrigation. I wheelbarrowed loads of rocks while my teammates collected piles. Together we planted, harvested, washed, weeded, and shipped out tens of thousands of pounds of produce across the island. We grew 10 kinds of salad greens, big beautiful beets, carrots, turnips, radishes, mangos, papayas, edible flowers, edible tree leaves, and more. We cared for 400 chickens and a small herd of sheep. We trapped wild pigs. We threw a farm festival and shared our mission with our fellow farmers. Our days were good.

Eventually it was time to go back to Magic where the extreme difference in lifestyle was stark and depressing. I took flights to convention centers and spent many weekends indoors. I stayed in random cities where no food was growing. I spent more of my time sitting on the computer. For what? I was grateful for the platform to share, but was this the most important thing I could be doing with my life? What was the point of all this? I wanted to go back to organic farming and I wanted to do it full time. But I wasn't one to quit and I was obligated to make it to the rest of the events for the year. I was set to take off for another months long trip through Europe.

Luckily, the choice was made for me. The way things shook up I wasn't invited to the events like I thought. The tournament lifestyle was high variance and just like it started, it finished. While it would end the lifestyle I had been living, I immediately recognized this as a blessing. My business would live on, but I wouldn't have to fly around to competitions anymore. I had gone too far down the wrong path and I was freed to start over with new commitments. I could do what I wanted, and what I wanted to do was go back to the land. Luckily, I was still in a position to pay to work, and they were happy to take me back. I picked up my stuff and moved to Hawaii to become a full-time farmer.

I am very lucky to be writing this from the farm right now. I had to accomplish my goals in time to realize there was so much more to life. I had to realize what I was missing and go search for it. I had to draw the right card at the right time. I had to find the right place at the right time. I had to meet the right people at the right time. I had to have a side business to afford the move. I had to be freed from my obligations. I had to have the physical health and diligence to perform on the farm. Everything had to line up, and it did. I'm very grateful to be here. And I realize a lot of people are waking up and want my spot. I'll tell you, we don't have to compete, there is still plenty of room on the land. I am happy to help you with that.

The life is good. We work on something we believe is extremely important. We work hard from sunrise to sunset. We live on the land. We work on the land. We harvest our own food and share it together. The sun shines down on us. The wind blows on us. The rain pours on us. The plants are happy. The animals are happy. The people are happy. It's hard work and a huge commitment, but we have community. We have mission. We have purpose. We have certainty. This is the life right here.

You don't have to travel the world to find it. You don't have to move to California or Hawaii. It's not in any one place. It's on the land all around you. It's in the community garden right down the street. It's on the rooftop in the city. It's on the local farm nearby. It's on your back porch. If you decide to search for it, you'll find it- right under your feet.

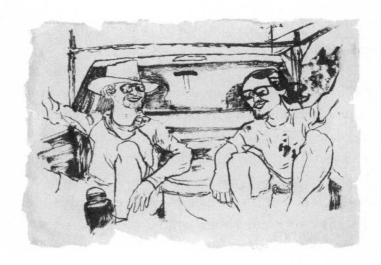

Tommy

Tommy finally snapped. He quit his job, sold his things, gave his dog to family, broke up with his girlfriend, and moved out of state to become an organic farmer. Like many millennials, he took out a massive student loan debt to go to college and in return got a miserable office job to try to pay it off. His screen savers were beautiful landscapes that he could at best vacation to a few short weeks of the year. But at 30 years old, he had finally paid off his debt and stashed enough cash to make a play for The Food Life.

For the first time in decades the average age of farmers is getting younger. Older farmers are passing on, and young people are excited to take their place. We've seen a massive citification of human life since the industrial revolution. I doubt we'll see a full flight to farm reversal, but there's a real trend happening here. Young people see organic farming as a relatively desirable lifestyle. There are millions of Tommys out there, currently grinding away at their nine to five keyboard job.

Millennials have become skeptical of the corporate dream. Or, maybe they've seen the truth.

Looking down the end of the tunnel there's not even a pension there. Just a shitty lifestyle stuck indoors, with plenty of related health problems, and a yearning to be anywhere outdoors. Meanwhile, during lunch break, or probably right in the cubicle, they're on their phone, on Instagram, looking at that one friend who's out on the farm in some exotic destination. They're holding baby animals, eating delicious foods, working in a beautiful landscape, and they look healthy and happy. Anyone would be envious.

If anything will lead young people back to the land, it's social media. It looks great on picture. It looks great on video. Because it's great in real life. Taking a picture of your coffee mug on your desk is only so inspiring. But a bunch of freshly pulled carrots makes a beautiful picture. That rack of bananas is going to garner a lot of likes, and it's also going to be tasty. Young farmers on social media are the marketing force that will accelerate the movement of young people from corporate jobs back to the farmland. It's going to happen, whether it pays well or not.

Of the young organic farmers around me, most of them are either ok with having less money, saved money like Tommy, or work a second job to pay for the first. I came into the game with an online side business, which let me work for free for a year before finally getting paid the lowest hourly wage I had in ten years. But I didn't care, because it's not about the money. We are rewarded in other ways.

If money was not a problem, what would you do? At first you might do nothing, but then you would get bored. You might start traveling, but after a few years of leisure while your friends work you would probably get bored again and want to get back to work. And there's a good chance you would turn to some kind of farming. The farm is more and more an end goal. It's something you do once you've secured the bag and can execute on any option.

It's all about lifestyle. You throw any animal in a cubicle with instructions to sit still and look at the monitor and that animal will get antsy, no matter how many years of "education" prepared them for this. Growing food is the new cool thing to do. If people aren't quitting out and going back to the land, they're starting to garden, plant trees, and volunteer at the local farm. Professional by day, farmer by weekend is a growing trend. Anything to get offline and get outside for a minute. People can't take it anymore, especially with the knowledge of what's possible out there.

Organic farmers are the new rock stars. This is the new lifestyle so many people want. It's becoming more obvious that the glamorous lifestyle of performers has its problems, with so many young stars dying from substance abuse and suicide. You see the pro athletes who get traded to some shithole city away from their families, have short careers, and go on with injured bodies for the rest of their lives. If you want to aspire to that, go ahead. Someone should, and it can be a great lifestyle. But more people can be farmers, and it seems that the reality is it can be even better. We talk about it on the farm. We're regular people that don't care to be rich or famous, and we don't want to go back to the corporate life either. More young people will come back to farming, but there's no chance Tommy is going back to the office.

Paige

When Paige graduated high school, she wasn't sure what she wanted to do. Unlike Tommy and many of her peers who took out debt to go to University where they hoped to figure it out later, she decided she would save her money and go on a volunteer farming adventure instead. She loved the work, the nature, the growth of baby plants and animals, the wind, the sun, the mountains, and the food. Within a year she had put in a thousand hours running farmer's markets and was growing and selling her own flowers. Many of her peers were going to school, studying, and partying, with the idea that they would figure it all out in time. At 19, skipping college and going directly to The Food Life, Paige was way ahead of the game.

A lot of young people are waking up to the University scam. Sure, for some people who want to be doctors or lawyers, college actually is necessary. For some people it's a great call. But for many others it's not. A few decades ago, you could pay for college working part time, and it gave a significant edge on the job market. Today college is not at all affordable and it doesn't guarantee much of anything. For many people it's a four-year delay under a lifetime of crippling debt.

Unlike Paige, Jamie decided to go to an expensive college even though she wasn't sure what career she wanted to pursue. She ended up gravitating towards The Food Life. She enjoyed the work, the lifestyle, and the people. Eventually she was living the dream managing a small farm where I met her as a volunteer. While she's passionate for farming and good at her job, the pay gives little hope of paying off her debt. For those saddled with debt, the financial weight disincentivizes having children. A worthy sacrifice for her to do the work she loves, but also a cautionary tale for young people. There is a more direct path to the land.

I'm happy that I finally discovered the agriculture lifestyle at 25, but I would have preferred a seven-year head start by choosing a different route. I went to an in-state college, fortunately staying out of debt, and while I worked hard in and out of school, none of it led me to the work I would eventually be doing. I didn't go to graduation, never collected my diploma, and haven't made a resume since. I earned work through meeting people and demonstrating my value. I got paid by marketing services and making calls. I got jobs by showing up and volunteering for free long enough until they had to pay me. The world just doesn't work the way my guidance counselor advised.

You won't figure out what you want to do with your life by theorizing. You must try things. You can't just see it on TV or read about it in books. You have to get your hands dirty. You have to eat from the buffet of life to learn what tastes best for you. We see too many casualties of the conventional route. The world has changed, and while she chose a different path, I think Paige is right on.

Takuya

Takuya, a Japanese professional actor, came to Hawaii with this girlfriend for a three-week yoga retreat. On Tuesdays the yoga group would come out onto the farm to enjoy nature and get their hands dirty. I met Takuya on the farm. He was covered with tattoos, which is really unusual in Japanese culture, but he assured me he was not a Yakuza gang member. They helped us harvest roots and work on clearing rocks from a new field. Takuya fell in love with the work immediately, and upon returning to Japan, immersed himself in agriculture. In his new life his social media became all farm life- transplanting baby kale, petting sheep, and laughing with the other farmers. After three months of farming in Japan he came back with his girlfriend to work with us for another three months, for no pay, purely for love of the work. While riding in the back of the farm truck with a harvest of freshly pulled roots, Takuya told me that farming, not acting, is the "Ichiban" (number one) job.

We tend to romanticize lifestyles that are high paying, high status, and high freedom. A lot of young people would like to be professional competitors, professional musicians, professional actors or now professional social media influencers. Maybe money will buy happiness, but if not then attention and freedom surely will. Unfortunately, for most humans this is myth. Money's correlation to happiness doesn't extend far beyond providing food and shelter. Too much attention causes anxiety. Freedom from an awful job is nice, but unlimited travel and leisure causes disconnection and depression. Society has foisted the wrong goals on us. The truth is work with high meaning brings the best chance for happiness.

We don't work primarily for money. We worked for millennia before the invention of money. Most rich people continue to work. Most early retirees restart their lives with a second career. We work for meaning. The goal isn't to be free from commitment. The goal is to be free to choose to commit to things we feel are very meaningful.

For me, Tommy, Takuya, Paige, Jamie, and I, farming is high meaning work. We're willing to give up a lot. We could be making more money doing something different. We could be traveling the world. We could be in the spotlight. But we don't think that's the best life. We enjoy The Food Life. We like to work outside with nature. We like to sweat and get our hands dirty. And most importantly, we know our work really matters.

Tai

Tai Lopez, more than anyone else, got me interested in farming. I was visiting my parents in Seattle on my way back from another trip abroad and was continuing back to California in the morning. I felt disoriented, lost, and unsure of what to do next with my life and why. Looking for direction and inspiration I went to YouTube and searched Tony Robbins. I never made it to Tony after a Tai Lopez video ad popped up first.

"Here in my garage, just bought this new Lamborghini here. It's fun to drive up here in the Hollywood hills. But you know what I like more than materialistic things? KNOWLEDGE! In fact, I'm a lot more proud of these seven new bookshelves that I had to get installed to hold two thousand new books that I bought. It's like the billionaire Warren Buffett says, "the more you learn, the more you earn."

Now maybe you've seen my TEDx talk where I talk about how I read a book a day. You know, I read a book a day not to show off it's again about the knowledge. In fact, the real reason I keep this

Lamborghini here is that it's a reminder. A reminder that dreams are still possible, because it wasn't that long ago that I was in a little town across the country sleeping on a couch in a mobile home with only 47 dollars in my bank account. I didn't have a college degree, I had no opportunities.

But you know what? Something happened that changed my life. I bumped into a mentor. And another mentor. And a few more mentors. I found five mentors. And they showed me what they did to become multimillionaires. Again, it's not just about money, it's about the good life; health, wealth, love and happiness. And so I record a little video, it's actually on my website, you can click here on this video and it'll take you to my website where I share three things that they taught me. Three things that you can implement today no matter where you are."

A lot of people would have "SCAM" alarm bells going off in their head, but I didn't. I was searching for a teacher and here he was. I clicked onto his site and enrolled into his 67 Steps course for $67. Over the next two months I listened to him every day, did exercises, and journaled. I started reading more. I cleaned up my habits. I found some direction and was running with it.

Of Tai's millionaire mentors, it turned out the first was Joel Salatin of Polyface Farms. I happened to be reading about Joel's Farm in Michael Pollan's "The Omnivore's Dilemma." Joel is a celebrity in the integrity farming world and Tai was his first apprentice. Instead of going to college, Tai had gone to live with Joel on the farm after high school, then worked on farms in Amish communities for several years. Later he continued his agritourism to New Zealand where he checked out other kinds of farming. Later he moved back to the city for night club business, became a certified financial planner, got into Google ads, started investing in companies, moved to the Beverly Hills, then finally burst onto the scene with his "Here in my garage" video and a ten-million-dollar ad budget. Tai goes on and on about his time on the farm in search of The Good Life, how happy the people are, how much he learned, how it set him up for success, and how it was some of his best times. I had never had that hands-on experience and I wanted it for myself, so I went out in search of it. Within a month I was volunteering at the community garden, then the city farm, and within two years living and working on an organic farm full time.

Tai still regularly visits Joel, the Amish, and has a ranch out in Virginia where they use horse power to plow their fields. It's a crazy story. Rags to riches, and he recommends riches. But farm life to city life? Better to be a rich farmer I suppose. Few people actually get to experience both sides of the coin. Pay careful attention to the final choices of those who do.

Tai Lopez talks of "health, wealth, love, and happiness". These things are not to be obtained. They are to be grown. He recommends to "Bloom where you were planted," but for me I think a scattered seed may need to search and relocate. Whatever, wherever. The point is you need roots in the ground to ever fruit. You need roots for years, decades even, to bloom-. You need roots with the people around you, so you can really trust them, understand them, and grow together.

"*The Good Life*" was a book by Helen and Scott Nearing, a couple who left the city to farm in the woods of Vermont. They built a life together with nature, the land, and with the community around them. Things were simpler, and they were happier. Decades later they took the time to write about it. I'm sure this book crossed Tai's path in his quest to read a book a day. Health, wealth, love, and happiness- everything Joel Salatin and the Amish possessed. These are rich people. More evidence that The Good Life is actually The Food Life.

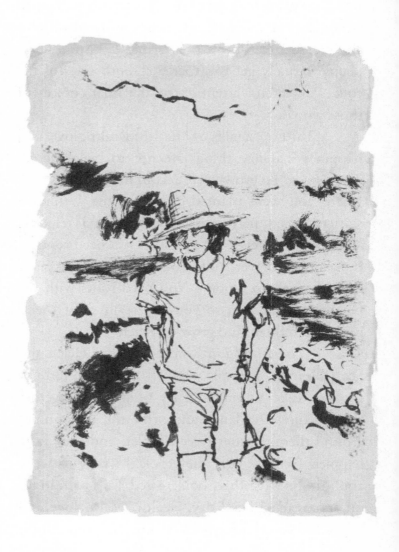

The Good Life

The Good Life is very simple. It's in the small things. The obvious things. Good food. Good people. Good work. Good community. Good missions. Good tastes, sights, sounds, smells, and sensations. Good health. A good laugh. A good night's sleep. Good days. Just enough money to not have to worry much. Sunshine on your cheeks, soil between your toes. Clean air. A sprinkle of rain and wind in your hair. Birdsong and trees rustling on the ears. Swimming in the oceans and lakes. Feeding the animals. Playing with children. Sticking with something until you succeed and celebrating the fruits of our labor all together.

It's unfortunate that so few of us get to experience The Good Life, but it's not because it's extremely difficult to attain. It's because society foists the wrong goals on most of us. They tell us to sit still, be quiet, keep going, graduate, get a good job, dress a certain way, act a certain way, go to the gym, create an appearance on social media, have a certain kind of relationship, accrue material things together, and go on vacation from life every once in a while. Some of these things are nice, but they make the wrong target.

Where's the emphasis on good days? Community? Being able to express yourself as a human animal?

It's no one's fault. There's no conspiracy. But there is a broken system and a lot of lost people. Big marketing and advertising are distracting us from what matters. Most people are off pursuing the wrong goals. There aren't enough people living The Good Life to teach it. There aren't even enough people pursuing The Good Life to share it. But there are a few. It's an old movement that has nearly died, but it's coming back, and I believe will grow. The people who have it are sharing it and you know it when you see it. You can only sit in a job you don't like looking at the wonderful world out there through screen savers and social media for so long before snapping off and going for it yourself.

I believe it's possible for anyone. You don't need a million dollars. You don't need a ton of things. You don't need to move to Hawaii. You don't have to travel 365. You don't have to look a certain way. You don't have to show up for a job you don't believe in. All you have to do is pursue The Good Life and the stuff that makes up good days, weeks, months, years, and decades. It's simple things that are freely available to you everywhere in the world.

I recommend you follow the food trail. Find out where the good stuff is coming from. Go to the source. The people closest to the best food are certainly on to something. Go there. Eat the food. Get involved. Volunteer. Enjoy the sights, sounds, and smells. You won't find The Good Life overnight. But I'm telling you, if you try for it, it can happen faster than you think.

Farmily

It's good to have a big family. An extended kin network. Multiple generations living close with brothers, sisters, mothers, fathers, daughters, sons, uncles, aunts, nephews, and nieces. People who you instinctively love and care for. It is good to share blood with people so you can step up and take care of each other when it matters most. With more family comes more security. But most of us do not have this. We may have a strong relationship with our parents and siblings, but there's a good chance it's a small family and you don't live that close to many relatives.

In the old times, we lived closer to kin. We grew up in villages with neighbor villages. But modernization, technology, and cheap ease of travel caused people to scatter across the globe. Immigration took off. Most people don't live in ancestral grounds. More and more people are off on their own with few or no family. People get lonely.

If you feel something is missing, but you're not sure what it is, it could be this. It could be a lot of things, but why not more family? Consciously, or subconsciously, we seek more family. We make friends, we go to events, we join groups and clubs, we volunteer. We seek deeper relationships.

I love my parents and my brother, but they live far away from me. They live far away from where their parents and siblings lived. We scattered. I made friends, but I was missing a family. I made some brothers through competition, but not enough to fill the void.

Young farmers find their family on the farm. The Good Life working together with family. Farmers coming together to help each other out. Companions toil in the fields and share our bread. Through blood, sweat, and tears, we show up to harvest. We live together, we struggle together, we celebrate the fruits of our labor together. Teammates become brothers, sisters, parents, children. We might not share blood, but we become surrogate family.

I found my family on the farm. My mother didn't have me until her 40s. I remember her asking me if I wanted a sister. I would have liked a little sister. I think she tried, but it didn't happen. But many years later, I found my little sister on the farm. And much more. This is deeper than blood. This is farmily.

The Modern Homestead

Ned and Devin got a small piece of land outside of the city about three years ago. In the first year they mostly assessed and planned, but also got a flock of chickens and started harvesting eggs. In the second year they got electricity, built a well for water, and got the land ready for planting. In the third year they got a dog, pigs, ducks, took responsibility for their neighbors' goats, and planted a food forest. A lot could happen in the fourth year, including building a house and moving onto the property to live. It's exciting.

The farm has been funded by off farm work in the city, which is the norm for modern homesteading. It makes sense financially. In the early stages a farm is a massive money sink, and at this scale it will probably never be particularly profitable. It makes sense socially. It can take decades to build a community, and right now it's just the two of them. It's more about the lifestyle- the pleasure of feeding the birds, feeding the hogs, feeding the dog, feeding the goats, watching the crops grow, harvesting, and eating together.

Ideally homesteading is something you do with your family. It's a social living arrangement that mixes work, play, and food. It's probably not something you'd want to do alone. Farming is a hard life for a hermit. It gets lonely. And it's difficult to do alone. It gets exponentially easier with a team on the same page.

If you don't have a partner, find people to work with who are already doing it. Once you meet the key personnel you can start your own thing, but you don't have to. Intentional community farming is a new way to homestead that accommodates the modern reality that a lot of people are missing family support because of the immigration shuffle. Farmily is family.

Homesteading is a pretty nice living arrangement if you can manage it. You have your family and your pets in your cozy modern house, eat the fruits of your labor, surrounded by plants that you grew, animals that you care for, nestled quietly in the woods. If you could snap your fingers and make it happen, most people probably would. But most people don't know about it. Even if they did, it's not nearly that easy. It takes a lot of hard work, on and off the farm, but it's something that people are still working for.

Food

Lifestyle

A Day in the Life of a Farmer

We start before dawn. It's dark, but you can hear birds singing and roosters crowing. We split up for chores, cleaning up the wash station, feeding the animals, watering the greenhouse, writing orders up on the board. I scrounge our shelves and bins for overripe fruit for the pigs and collect greens for the sheep. We organize and head out to the fields for today's harvest, snipping salad, pulling and topping roots, collecting kale and chard leaves, bundling herbs, picking eggplant and fruit. We watch the sun rise over the mountains. Once we have the weights we need, we load up, head back, and log our haul. On a great day we might harvest 350 pounds of salad, 200 pounds of carrots, beets, turnips or radishes, 40 pounds of kale and chard, 40 pounds of herbs, 20 pounds of eggplant, 20 pounds of luau leaves, 10 pounds of papaya, and maybe some fennel, leeks, and purplettes. Truly a bounty. We get the roots soaking with water, move the greens to the fridges, wipe the mud off our shoes, and head to breakfast.

For breakfast, I have a heaping pile of our green, purple, and red salad with mild baby kale, lettuce, and mizuna, spicy tatsoi, garnet, rain, and streaks, bitter amaranth leaves, dressed in olive oil. I slice some of our seasonal fruit. It could be banana, mango, drangonfruit, watermelon, orange, jabong, coconut grapefruit, pineapple, passionfruit, guava, sapodilla, jackfruit, or soursop. A fruit heaven. I toast a piece of organic bread, top it with butter and our eggs, and wash it all down with coffee and our hibiscus herbal cooler. I know, it's a historically great breakfast. Few people have ever eaten this good. Before returning to work I take a few minutes to make a phone call, write, record a video, stretch, or play the piano.

Next comes the washing. We fill eight sinks with water, pour in the salad, and pull out weeds, bugs, and boogery leaves. I collect the sorted leaves in drying baskets, spin them through a machine, and sort them into labeled tubs to be moved back into the fridge to preserve maximum freshness. Someone sprays the roots clean, I help prepare for farmer's market. Local sellers come in with their backyard fruit for us to resell. The eight different salad leaves are mixed. Produce is bagged, and as orders are fulfilled they get crossed of the board. One person goes out to feed chickens while someone else goes to water the greenhouse. We go to lunch.

For lunch, our farm to table café serves us vegetable soup, a spicy arugula salad topped with shaved radish or shredded carrots with a green herb dressing, a starchy local breadfruit, organic pasta, potato, or rice, with maybe some organic chicken for protein. I salt heavily and wet it with chili pepper water. If I want even more nutrition I might make a smoothie with frozen banana, seasonal fruit, turmeric, moringa, soursop, chia, flax, cacao, and honey or go out for some fresh caught fish. We break for the heat of the day when the sun is at its strongest, and I take the time to nap, read, write, record, make calls, do laundry and clean, or play in the ocean.

We return in the afternoon to organize, then split up. One person goes to market, one person goes on deliveries, one person goes on tours, one person goes on tractor work, one person weed whacks, two people go to plant seeds, and a team goes out to handle the most pressing issue- prepping the newest field, breaking down the oldest field, applying organic fertilizer, hula-hoeing small weeds from the new root field, hand weeding large weeds from the maturing root field, or transplanting from the greenhouse. I collect unused root tops and B-grade salad leaves from earlier in the day for the sheep, and run by the café to grab slop for the pigs. Someone splits off to water the fields and orchards. If it's a Friday we might plant trees, prune the orchard, work on animal shelters, or slaughter and butcher meat. I lead the sheep out to pasture and daydream about lambs weeding the orchard and pigs turning our old root fields. As the sun sets the mountains are illuminated with a golden glow. Dusk comes, and we head back.

For dinner in the café, we are treated with more vegetable soup- a rich orange carrot, vibrant red beet, creamy ulu, or menagerie of turnips and radishes. This time our salad is stir fried and topped over an ulu mash or cheesy pasta. If we're lucky we'll eat our own lamb or pork, but more often a local beef, venison, or wild caught fish topped with dill or lilikoi sauce. Sometimes we'll face the dilemma of organic pork or chicken from Costco, or forego meat altogether for the day. If I want an after-dinner snack, I'll turn to some trail mix featuring local macadamia nuts or grab a frozen banana. After dinner, I'm physically exhausted and have the energy only to clean myself up and lay down to browse and read before sleeping like a log.

It doesn't stop on the weekends. We have volunteer day, farmer's markets, and farm to table events. The animals still need to eat, and the fields still needs watering. Weeds keep growing. I like to take it easy on Sunday, but there is always work that could be done. In many parts of the world, the farm slows down with the turn of the season. As harvest finishes, the days get shorter, the weather is too cold to plant, and there is time to read, reflect and write. But if you farm in the tropics, it's a 365-day growing season and the work never stops. Personally, I found the seasonal lag boring and feel lucky to work on the land year-round.

Our lives as farmers are far above the historical norm. We grow a dizzying variety of foods and have access to worldwide markets. We eat extremely varied diets. Although we do specialize, we get to work varied jobs to support so many different crops, animals, and programs. Our agricultural ancestors ate only a few staple crops year-round and had more repetitive work lives centered around the same few crops. If our crops are wiped out by a weather disaster, we can go to the store, while our ancestors may have starved. This is not the same drudgerous farming that our great-great-grandparents fled for city jobs. Modern organic farming is a whole new paradigm that is richer than ever before possible. For those of us young folks returning to the land, it's not just a return to past ways, but reimagining and creating a better future.

Even amongst modern farmers, we live extremely good lives. Our various diets and jobs come with a large team with low turnover. We've inherited the infrastructure of a 40-year-old nonprofit organization- knowledge, programs, buildings, equipment, and land. The local governments are on our side. I know that you can build something like this, but I also know how long it takes, and have little desire to try to start from scratch. Farming is always a grind but starting a new one comes with a lot of uncertainty and oftentimes lonely work before a permanent team is comes together. But the ultimate potential is higher than it's ever been, and if there's one trait farmers have in common it's the ability to imagine the future and manifest it.

Wherever, whenever, and however you're farming, our lives share a few important things in common. We watch the sunrise; we watch the sun set. We feel the beat of the seasons and the breeze of the trees. We work with other life. We cocreate with nature. We labor. We do the work we have time to do, with long lists of work we'd like to do. Our backs and knees ache. We imagine a better future and build for it. We harvest and eat the fruits of our harvest. We go to sleep easy at the end of the day, dream of plants and animals, and rise early to run it back again tomorrow.

The Steward's Oath

As steward of the land it is my responsibility to work with integrity, love, and devotion to regenerate the Earth, bring healthy soil, rear happy animals, and share abundant food with other humans to help bring them health and happiness. My obligation goes beyond the farm, my job, the business, the animals, and the people. This work is cocreation with God, mother nature, the Universe, whatever you want to call it. I work with her resources, under her sun, feeling her breeze, taking her weather as it comes, with the body she gifted me, reaping her rewards. I do not take this lightly, and I will do the most I can. Thank you for this opportunity.

Whether big acreage or one potted plan on the porch, growing food is a special responsibility. With it comes stewardship. You become the guardian of the soil, the bugs, the plants, the fruits, the animals, and the eaters of the food. Failure to maintain your responsibility, through neglect or poor practices, results in death, erosion, and degeneration. If you do not provide water, the plant will die, the bugs will die, the soil will die, the humans will not be fed. After the decision to become steward, it is your continuing duty to protect and care for your charge.

We live in a society with less and less stewardship. Humans have uprooted and lost connection to their land. The temporary nature of modern lifestyle disincentivizes people from fully investing in where they are. Why would I care for a tree when I might move at the end of my lease and I can't take it with me? Private and public property laws cause people to believe problems outside their home aren't their problems. They say if each person swept their porch we would have a clean society. But what if everyone came out together and started cleaning garbage from our streets, parks, rivers, streams, and oceans? If we collectively took responsibility for our world, not in the legal sense, but as a sacred stewardship appointment from God, imagine the results. We can protect it. No more needless pollution and destruction of our environment and lands. Regeneration of the soil and return of biodiversity. It is our duty. This is the steward's oath.

Living Together

Modern societal lifestyle is weirdly separated. You live in your house or apartment with walls and fences between your neighbors. You may or may not know them, but you probably aren't friends, don't work together, and don't share with each other. Instead you take a car and drive to your work or school on separate land with separate people. You're probably friends with some of them, but maybe not even that. The food you buy from the store has no connection to your work or living. The gym you visit is also in a different place with different people. Your friend group is also different and the venues you visit together are again different. Every component of modern life is separate from the others. It allows more anonymity, but at the cost of depth.

Community living is integrated all together. Your fences are around the community, not between individuals. You know and love your neighbors. You live on or near the land you work. You work with people you live with. You eat and play with your teammates and neighbors. You own your own stuff, but you share with each other. Everything bleeds into everything else. The magic is in the edges. You may

53

have the option to leave if you want, but you might just want to hang around and go deeper. You have very little anonymity and that forces you to be more accountable and responsible for your actions. You can't burn bridges, instead you have to repair and live with each other. Community lifestyle is no longer the norm, but it feels normal because for the vast history it has been normal.

Nowadays very few people are even exposed to community living, and if they are, they may think of them as culty. It's easier to understand when you realize humans have been living in community villages and nomadic tribes for most of our history. The advent of private property and government restrictions slowly made it abnormal. The nuclear family is relatively new. Most governments do not want their people congregating on the land together which is why in many cases it is illegal. We feel little choice but to build walls and fences between each other.

If you ever feel isolated in modern society, this is probably why. I feel you. You may have great friends and family, but something still feels missing socially. I felt lonely too. When I first heard of "intentional communities", the idea immediately made sense, and I wanted in. I began to seek them out. I saw a few that worked well and a key commonality between them was growing a portion of their own food together and sharing it. The integrated life is all about food. One road led me to organic farming, and now that I'm here it's hard to ever imagine going back.

For you, The Good Life might be the integrated farm life. If it is, follow the food trail to your nearest community gardens and organic farms. You'll be able to find it there. But this isn't for everyone and it won't just happen overnight. In the short term the goal should be to bridge the gap between the separated parts of your life. How can you merge your living, your work, your play, your neighbors, your teammates, and your friends? It's not easy but there are a few things you can do. Invite your neighbors over for dinner. Go out to eat with your coworkers. Live closer to your work. Bring everybody together for a big potluck. Invite everyone around the food. If you build community, they will come. Almost everyone is looking for it, few have it, and even fewer realize they're missing it. But when they see it, they will know. When you invite them, they will want in. This is how you grow community. This is how you begin to live an integrated life.

Intentionally

I've lived in unintentional communities, from modern housing, to apartments, to dorms. But I've also lived in intentional communities. After experiencing the difference, it's hard for me to go back to what most of modern society is doing. There's something about bringing people together on the land on purpose that simply feels normal. That's because intentional communities are closer to the villages and tribes we've lived in for most of our history as humans.

An intentional community is when people come together on purpose, live together, choose each other, share the land, and develop structure to the lifestyle and an intentional connection to the people around them. It could be shared housing, or it could be individual housing with shared eating facilities. There could be shared duties and weekly events. It's pretty different than a random assortment of people who just happen to live in the same place, who don't have a plan for living together, or intention on spending time with the group as a whole. There are many intentional communities, a few of them culty,

56

but many of which are built by regular people who have a vision of a better way of living.

We don't grow our best alone. We grow better together. We don't build our best alone. We build our best together in teams. That's the premise of intentional communities. It's a simple concept. The garden can be bigger and better, the meals can be tastier and better prepared. We can throw better events to meet more interesting people. A single person on their own can only do so much, but a whole clan can build an astounding life together where most of the good things you need are right around you.

The actual truth is that we've been living in intentional communities for most of history. A handful of families would gather together and decide to do the best they can. They make up some rules and customs for living life and how people will come and go. They might live in their own houses, but if there are fences it's around the community rather than separating it. As people moved more and more to industrialized cities, individuals and small families had their umbilicals cut and moved about with relative anonymity, without an extended clan or group.

You'd think more people would still be living this lifestyle, and I think more people would go back if they knew and thought they could. Unfortunately, there are even governmental obstacles and restrictions around living on agricultural land, such as limits on how many people can live together in certain places. I'm not sure how this helps people, but in many places it's the law. It doesn't mean it's impossible, as there are workarounds and permits to make it all happen.

If you feel a bit lonely in the modern world, that's entirely normal because of the disconnect between modern and ancient living. You may be missing your tribe. You could find it living together with other people. It's probably worth trying it first before going all in and trying to create your own. Some people have become wired for the cities and prefer the more anonymous living style with fewer rules. But a lot of people thrive when living in groups of other people. Go for a search on the internet where you might be something popping up in your area. They probably grow food too. It's worth exploring to see what you find.

Life on the Edges

In nature, the boundary between different ecological environments is ripe with increased biodiversity and abundance. This is called the edge effect. For instance, the edge between freshwater and saltwater is the salmon breeding ground. The edge between the forest and the river is where the bears go. Where the ocean meets land, where the prairie meets forest, where the city meets country is where all the action is at. Wherever you go, there's more life on the edge. This goes beyond nature.

When it comes to farming, we want the advantages and the security of the edge effect. A monoculture farm has no inner edges. It has limited biodiversity and is at risk of a single disease or pest wiping out everything. Monoculture farmers turn to increasing pesticides, herbicides, and GMO crops for protection. But in organic and biodynamic farming, the edge offers all the protection needed.

If you think of the farm as a living organism, you want the security of increased biodiversity, and you want the increased biodiversity that comes with many edges. More edges mean more predator insects to balance pest populations, more barrier plants to slow the spread of disease, and more productive crops. Understory trees do better with overstory trees. Climbing vine plants do better with a trellis to grow on. Lining rows with flowering plants and fruit trees can attract the bugs you need to keep everything in balance.

When it comes to overall health of the organism, the more edges the better. How do the sheep intersect with the garden? How do the pigs intersect with the kitchen? How do the bees interact with the flowers? More edges mean more action. There is more complexity, but that is a fine price to pay for health and security.

The edge effect goes even deeper. Like a healthy farm, The Food Life is all about the edge effect. Monocropping corn with machines doesn't sound like all that great of a lifestyle. But working with animals, kids, and food has something special at the intersection. Living at the edge of food, community, and charity is a wonderful place to be. The more programs, missions, organizations, and food products, the richer, more abundant, more fun, more exciting. The Food Life lives on the edge of food, work, and mission.

The modern lifestyle is an example of what happens when you take away most of the edges. Think about what happens when you separate education from work, work from play, work from home, and work from exercise. You end up with a lot of people who don't really like their work all that much. You have lives that are compartmentalized, isolated, and segregated. People get lonely and depressed. People fall through the cracks. But if you can bring it all together, what happens at the edge of work, play, home, and exercise? It can be a challenge making it all work together, but life always finds a way. Especially on the edge.

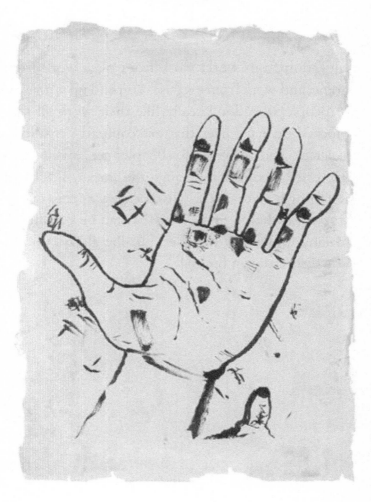

Work

You know you love your work when you do it for free and you could be making a lot more money doing something else. You know you love your work when you take on a second job to help pay for the first. You know you love your work when you look forward to getting up early on the weekends to get back at it. And when you love your work you put in more energy and attention. You care more about the process and the product. You do a better job and you get a better result.

There are a lot of reasons to be optimistic about the future. More and more young people are living out the scenario above. They're giving up high paying jobs in the city to work below minimum wage on organic farms. It's certainly not for money, so it must be out of love. And when you love the food you work on you get much better food. Society becomes healthier and more vibrant.

What should you do when you grow up? It's a tough question and hard to answer. Too few people love what they're doing to give good advice on this. They'll tell you to work for security, to work for stability, and to work for money. They'll tell you not to work for love because it's unrealistic and you can't make a good living. They'll tell you that if you follow what you love, you'll end up hating the work and ruining it. But just because it didn't work for them doesn't mean it can't work for you. Let's try a new approach.

Work a lot. Try many different things. Listen to your feelings. What do you love doing? Who do you love and how can you help them? Where do you love being? What work do you find yourself doing in your free time? Go deeper towards those things. If you love your gardening hobby, perhaps your occupation should be an organic farmer. But it could be anything. That's the beauty. Whatever it is, find more reasons to love it, and pour in more of yourself into it. Society needs more loving farmers, but society needs more loving everything. We need our teachers, service workers, and professionals to work out of love. With more love comes more laughter, more smiles, more work, better work, better result, a better you, and a better society.

Pay Me in Food

Pay me in food, because that's what I'm going to spend my money on anyways. Let's cut out the middle man. It's nice to have some spending money but if you've got good food and a nice place to stay you've already got the essentials. What more do you need? So I'll volunteer my time for food, especially if it's freshly washed produce pulled straight from the ground. Even better if I helped with the seeding and weeding, and if we cook it up right there and eat it all together. Pay me in food and I'm good. A simple solution for the complex problem of work, food, and life.

I got to a point where I was spending half of my money on food. If I made more money, I spent more on food. I went organic, I went local, I went exotic, I went gourmet, and I went for the premium health supplements. I know you can relate when you tabulate your expenses for the month. Where is all my money going? Mostly on food, so I should start getting paid in it.

This is why voluntourism is soaring and why young people are leaving the city for the paradise of a better food life balance. It sucks to be in a rush between school and work just to eat fast food that you didn't help produce, didn't help prepare, and doesn't make you feel good after you eat it. I wanted a better way where I could spend more time with my food. Let me help hill that potato, harvest that potato, and by the way, you can just pay me with some of those potatoes, and also should we bake or fry these potatoes right now?

It wasn't too long ago when food was the most common form of payment. Modern cash currency only came along after the agricultural revolution so that non-food workers could trade for food. Money was essentially invented for buying food. Of course, there are other services you would like to spend money on, but food is the only one that is truly essential. Historically, food growers have the least need for money, because they're already paying themselves in food. Today you may be paying thousands of dollars just for a tiny studio apartment in the city, so you'd think you need to make a lot of money to have a decent life. But you could also be living and working on an organic farm, have all your food and housing provided, and live a great life with only a little spending cash. So if you had to pick only one, would it be money or food?

Pay me in food, but only the good stuff please. That's the whole point of going there to help grow it. If I'm going to eat it, I want it to be good and healthy. And if I'm going to work on it, I want to eat it too. We're not out here working for top ramen packets, although that can be tasty too. We want the freshest, the brightest colored, the most loved, and the tastiest. Give us that and keep your money. We've got all we need fam.

Volunteer Day

Volunteer day is the gateway drug. You wander in. You try it one time. You get hooked. You keep coming back. You forget life before volunteer day. Before you know it, you're running volunteer day, and you see the future farmer in the new recruits. It's a small thing that does a lot. It builds community. It connects growers with eaters and buyers. And it introduces farming to the next generation of professional growers.

I started with volunteer day on a community garden, then a city farm, then a nonprofit production farm. We planted, we weeded, we harvested, and we hung out with the animals. We shared our stories of how we got here. Some of us traveled from far away. We hung around to snack and chat and left with bags full of fresh produce. I couldn't wait to come back next week. And when I left, I couldn't wait to stumble on the next volunteer day in my travels. I would pass them on the street, walk in, and get my hands dirty. I met the same kind of people- my people. Within three years I ran my first volunteer day, promoted the event, invited people, planned the work, gathered the tools, set up the water and shade, directed and coordinated, and handed out the produce at the end. So many hands came together to work on the food.

If you work once for free, you probably like it. If you continue to work for free, you probably love it. Volunteer day is trying it before buying it. If you keep coming back and laboring your time, you know this is it. This is your tribe, these are your people, this is your land, this is what you're supposed to be doing. Volunteers are happier. They know what makes them happy, and they make sure to keep doing it. Over time long term volunteers become professionals, except they skip the resumes, the application process, and the interviews. They gradually grow into the work. It's how I entered The Food Life, and I'm in good company.

I went searching for volunteer day, and I recommend the same for you. It's the entrance into a whole different world, with everything based around food. The work has everything to do with food, the pay has everything to do with food, the lifestyle has everything to do with food, the community has everything to do with food. It's a true food party, and everyone wants to be there, because we all chose to show up when we didn't have to. Ask around, use the internet, pick up the phone and call. It could be happening in the garden down the block, or on the secret farm down the road. You might be lucky enough to stumble past it like I did, but you will also probably have to go searching like me too.

Go to enough volunteer days and it will eventually be time for you to run your own. It's a chance to get a lot of work done in a short period of time. Many hands make light work. It's all about sharing and inviting. You invite the volunteers into your space, onto your land, into your work, to smell your garden, to taste your food, to meet your friends, to try your way of life. Volunteer day is your main vein with the surrounding community. The markets, community supported agriculture programs, and deliveries make nice connection, but volunteer day is an exchange of blood. It brings more people into your tribe, into your life, who want in for the right reasons. So put up a poster, make a social media post, let your friends and their friends know about volunteer day. Run it religiously, every Wednesday, every Friday, every first Saturday, or whatever you can always show up for. Volunteer day is a small thing that changed my life forever, and it could change your life forever too.

Food Explorers

Our hunter-gatherer ancestors were relatively nomadic people. They went out in search of better food, sometimes for pleasure, and sometimes because of no other option. From the cradle of Africa, food explorers slowly crept across the globe, filling the Eurasian land mass, hunting mastodons as they crossed the Bering land bridge, and worked their way down to the tip of South America. Even with the development of agriculture, nomadic lifestyles continued. Herd societies moved from winter quarters to summer pastures. As human populations increased and private property was invented, people started to stay in one place to farm. But the legacy of food exploration still runs in our blood, and at times the itch comes out.

In the late 1800s there were only a few staple crops growing in the United States, and many of those were low in quality. It took USDA special agent Food Explorers who crossed the globe in steamships in search of better crops for plant introduction to get us to where we are today. Frank Meyer, of Meyer lemon fame, walked across China sending back 25,000 useful plants including apricots, soybeans, and gingko biloba. David Fairchild was on of the most traveled men of his time, introducing more than 200,000 exotic plants such as mangos, nectarines, dates, pistachios, garbanzo beans, kale, seedless grapes, and Bavarian hops. We have these men to thank for our diverse bounty of options today. Fairchild and Meyer were famous in their time. Many young people dream of traveling the world in search of food, just like them. And while special agent plant introducers are a relic of the past, there is a new path for young people to travel the world and eat the food.

In today's world, not a lot of young folks grow up thinking they want to be involved in farming. It's just not on our radar. But most of us have a desire to travel while we're young, for adventure, or to try out something different for a while. With most of the human population now coming from cities, the other place is the country, and that different lifestyle is farming. By searching for what's missing, more and more young people are turning to WWOOFing as their answer.

WWOOFing, or World-Wide Opportunities on Organic Farms, is a global work trade network that lets volunteers give their time in exchange for housing and meals, and lets organic farms get valuable labor for cheap. You may have friends who have used WWOOF to work with livestock in

Columbia, vineyards in Europe, or tropical fruits in Hawaii. For many it's a great solution for how to travel, adventure, and have amazing experiences without spending much money. But after trying The Food Life, some become enamored, while others have their perspective changed and just can't go back to the old ways.

A nice thing about volunteer farm opportunities is the gateway to just try it. Not every career works that way. You can't dabble in being a doctor. Worse, you might spend a decade working towards it only to discover you don't really enjoy it that much. But with volunteer farming you get to try it before you buy it. You might not like it, but at least you won't waste years and hundreds of thousands of dollars on education. And once your foot is in the door you might find that it's the perfect lifestyle for you.

Farming is one of a few trades that while modernized with technology is still frozen in the past in many ways. For most farmers, you just start farming. There's usually no resume submission process. You just show up, ask to help, and start working. And like any ancient trade, you aren't going to be getting paid for a while, except in the literal fruits of your labor. The norm is to work for free, for food, or for housing for some time before eventually earning a paid position. It's a fine system. Apprentices don't necessarily deserve to be paid money. They consume time for their training and are paid in valuable, practical lessons.

If I had lived in the late 1800s, I would have liked to be a special agent Food Explorer like David Fairchild and Frank Meyer. Instead, I went with WWOOFing. I was a WWOOFer for a full year before signing a contract as a paid employee on an organic farm. It was a way to afford to live in a new part of the world and to do something totally different. I didn't know I would stay this long and that it would become my permanent work. But when you're excited to do something for free, you'll probably take the paid position if you can. For many like me, WWOOF starts as a food adventure but becomes the gateway into professional farming.

Food and Sleep

I used to think I was a genetic night owl, staying up past midnight staring into the lightboxes of my computer and phone. But when I moved to the country to be a farmer, I realized this was not the case. For the first time, my sleep was synced up with the true circadian rhythm-.I rose with the sun and set with the sun. In my past life in the city I had a hard time falling asleep at all, but now I had a hard time staying up past 9pm. My sleep dysfunction was caused by the ubiquity of artificial lighting and our cultural devaluation of sleep. These problems are rooted in our disconnection from food.

Our ancient ancestors didn't have much of a choice but to sleep when it was dark. Most of the animal world made this choice. Sleep was a chance to recharge, heal, grow, consolidate learning, and dream. There were no phone screens, flashlights, alarm clocks, street lamps, school bells, or punching into work. The invention of fire may have extended possible waking hours, but it wasn't until Thomas Edison's Electric Light Company in the recent past that electric lightning became available to everyone. And it wasn't until the past decade that the mobile phone as an entertainment device fell into our hands. We haven't had time to adjust, or sleep much.

Our culture is chronically sleep deprived, and many people are in denial about it. The effects of sleep deprivation, beyond poor performance, slow healing, stalled learning, and unregulated emotions, include increased fat storage and craving for junk foods. Too many of us stay up too late, eat awful food, feel like shit in the morning, and do it again that night. It's a vicious cycle that costs society in productivity and prudence. But who can we blame? It's not as simple as shutting off the phone. We miss the circadian-resetting sunrise while we're caught in traffic, school, or in office building. We're lucky if we get outside for lunch. If we work out at all, we get our heart pumping in the evening. And after fighting through traffic and eating dinner it's nice to escape and relax with modern technological luxuries. At some point, the sun set and we didn't even notice. The stars are drowned out by the glow of the city. The lights stay on.

I never slept so good until I became a farmer. I wake before dawn without an alarm. I catch the gaze of the sunrise coming over the mountains in the field. I soak up the morning sun and get my movement in early. I watch the sun set over the mountains or the ocean. It gets dark and I get tired. We head home to eat dinner, I turn off my phone, I read, look forward to the morning, and I fall sleep.

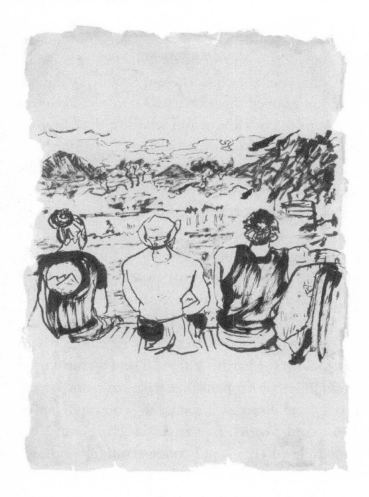

Earthing

Bare feet on soft earth. When's the last time you sunk your toes into the mud? When's the last time you gripped them on grass? If you're like most people in the modern world who live their lives on shoes and hard manmade surfaces, Earthing isn't something you do unless you're on vacation at the beach. If it feels normal, it's because it has been normal for millions of years. And the surprising thing is that studies indicate it's good for you too. The hippies might have been right about this one. Along with sunshine, clean air, clean water, nutritious food, and physical activity, Earthing could be essential for an optimal human life.

Earthing allows bare soles to connect with electrons on the Earth's surface. There is an electrical grounding that happens that seems to reduce stress, anxiety, and disease. It's something you could maybe understand with a science background, but something you can simply understand in your body when you do it. Bare feet, soft earth just feels good.

One problem with the modern world is our physical disconnection from the Earth. We spend a lot of time in shoes and a lot of time on concrete.

While concrete works great for car wheels, it isn't the best for our feet. Studies on elephants show a major increase in arthritis from increased time living on concrete. As the physical structure of our society has catered more towards automobiles, shoes have gone from thin animal skin sandals to thick rubber and synthetic soles. For most of us we might get to sink our feet into the sand every once in a while, but Earthing is no longer a part of our common lifestyle.

Increased Earthing was one of the attractions to the farm life for me. Our walkways and roads are grass, dirt, or gravel. The field rows are soft with damp soil. It's nice to kick off the shoes and connect our soles to Earth while we work with soil. The reality is you might have to deal with cold weather, fire ants, thorns, prickly carpet, staph, tropical skin diseases, disease-causing tics, and sun damage. In many regions it's sadly not that safe to go barefoot. Work boots can be necessary, depending on the situation. But show me a profession other than organic farming that gives you as much chance for to take your shoes off and walk on soft earth after a spring rain.

The solution isn't as easy as just kicking off your shoes and going for a walk. Our cities aren't designed for it. The few grass patches we have are usually reserved for dog poop. I wouldn't want to go barefoot there either. Cities aren't going to change their design with Earthing in mind, but maybe you can change yours.

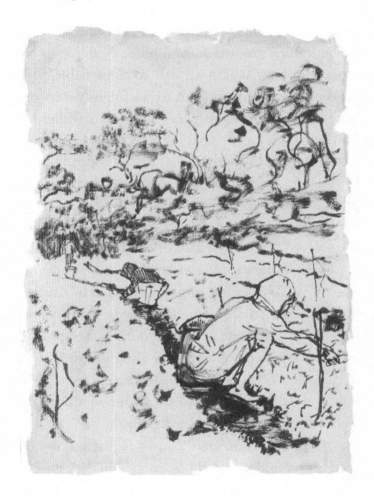

Farming in the City

The new trend for the super wealthy elite in Silicon Valley is backyard chickens. The answer for the working class in destitute areas of Detroit is reclaiming abandoned city blocks for community gardening. The rooftops over New York City are becoming covered with small grow operations. Microgreens are sprouting up under LED lights in basements. Container gardens are growing inside the city limits. Restaurants and cafes are planting herb gardens next to back patio seating. Intensive small grow operations are on the rise in cities. Today almost 20% of all food is now grown in cities.

While most of us now live in cities, most of our ancestors did not. City life is not for everyone. Some urban dwellers become bored and crazy and are compelled towards gardening as a satisfying life stabilizer. Others love urban living but feel that the farm life is even better. Some people are city people. Not everyone wants to move out to the country, but those same people still want to be around animals, plants, nature, outside, while watching the seasons turn.

The rules for farming in the city are flipped. It's not about efficiency, it's about intensiveness. You have to make the most out of the smallest plots. You have the time to micro manage each row, carefully applying composted kitchen scraps brought by community members. You can weed everything and leave no leaf behind. You might not have the biggest harvest, but with all that care you can grow some pretty incredible stuff to be sold at a premium.

For restaurants in the city, organic does matter, but local matters even more. Even organic salad doesn't hold or ship well. Ideally, it goes from harvest to customer's plate in only a few days. So trendy city restaurants would rather source from the block farm down the street than a large-scale operation in California. Organic certification is expensive, can take years, and doesn't guarantee the kind of care that intensive small-scale farming uses. Buyers want to meet the farmers and check out the operation for themselves.

Small intensive farms tend to get more yield per acre than big mechanized operations. The tradeoff is an increased need for labor. City farms are getting a lot of this labor through walk-on volunteers. Friends of farmers, people looking for a community, and future farmers looking to learn how it's done. I was all of these. If I left with a bag of stir fry greens and garlic that was great, but I was just happy to get my hands dirty.

People want to grow food, and they're going to grow food. It could be herbs on the window sill or potatoes from a sack of soil. It's not a trend promoted by the media or advertising norms. It's not for money or status. It comes from a seed deep inside us. Somewhere within there's an ancient desire to participate in the natural order of food growing. We've been doing this for eons, and we will be doing this for eons, whether in the country or the city.

Pros and Cons of The Food Life

I lived in a major city for 24 years, in a small city surrounded by farms for three years, and on a farm in the country since 2017. In that time alone I know that I will never go back to permanent city living and hope to live most of my life on biodiverse organic food farms. But as much as I romanticize The Food Life as The Good Life there are pros and cons to it, and it's not for everyone. Some people really thrive in the city, but you still never know until you try both.

First and foremost, you have the healthy lifestyle. Organic farming is probably the healthiest occupation, both on average and potential. You are spending most of your time moving outside. You are living close to the good food. You will be able to be healthier more easily. The downside of it is that you are dependent on your body for work and under risk of injury. If your body goes, you will be in trouble, and it's hard on the body. Many farmers get bad knees and bad backs from the physical labor. What do you do then? I think in many cases it is preventable. If you know how to protect your joints with proper movement you could age better than anyone. The health upside is very high.

The Food Life generally doesn't pay very well, in terms of money. There's a chance it does, but for most it is menial, below minimum wage, or subsidized by a second job online or in town. It's acceptable if you consider The Food Life also gives you a great lifestyle for low cost. You might not have to pay for food or rent. The days are good, the food is good, and the community has your back. You can have good security without a ton of money flowing. If you have food and company what else do you need?

It's not uncommon for farmers to struggle with loneliness. How many new people are you meeting? How many outsiders are coming onto the farm? How often are you getting off the farm and meeting people? You could find yourself alone or trapped with the few people you work with. Those relationships better be good! And they probably will be. All that time together means a chance for greater depth. You work together, you eat together, and you might live together too. You spend so much time together you can go deeper in relationships, and that is a major benefit of The Food Life.

You will be far from the action of town. If you crave crowds, strangers, shows, events, bars, parties, you may not have those luxuries on the farm. There's not so much going on out in the country aside from the occasional solstice, wedding, or harvest festival. You will get creative and have fun with your surroundings, which are beautiful. You might be far from the action, but you are close to the land, the food, the forests, the mountains, the water. It might not be noisy and exciting, but it sure is beautiful.

Farming can be really, really, really repetitive. You do the same things day after day, week after week, year after year. You make minor adjustments with the seasons, building off last year's lessons. The tasks can be a bit robotic and easy. You might get bored. But you will have time to think. And in that thinking time you will notice small changes. The trees grow day after day, week after week, year after year. New crops come and go. New fields sprout up. The animals put on weight and make babies. The landscape changes. You might be doing the same things, but over time you'll master those things and look back on big changes that have happened on the land

The farm lifestyle is not glamorous. Society appreciates it, when it's even aware of it, but does not glorify it. It's thought of something old people used to do, that now immigrants and machines do. You get sunburnt, wet, and dirty. It doesn't pay well, and it's not high status. But it's so important and you will be highly respected by people around you. Everyone eats food and appreciates their farmer. Society might not put you on the first tier, but you will get the satisfaction of rebellion. You didn't take the path that the system laid out for you, you did something more important, and you will be thanked.

At its worst, the farm lifestyle is backbreaking, poor, lonely, isolated, repetitive, and ignored. Historically farmers have struggled, and there's a reason many left the land to seek opportunities in the city. But it can be so, so good. At its best, it is physically liberating, a good living, with extra deep relationships, surrounded by beautiful scenery, participating in big changes, and comes with the satisfaction of knowing you sacrificed for the most important cause- good food. It's not a perfect life. That doesn't exist. It has its problems, but it's easily worth it. It was for your ancestors, and it may be for you too.

Food

Lives

Soil of the Earth

Did you know that one handful of healthy soil contains more microscopic life than there are humans on Earth? Like most people, I ate the food but didn't think about the soil. If you asked me, I knew it was dirt that plants grew from, but I didn't know about topsoil, humus, compost, or manure. I didn't have an opinion on fertilizers and herbicides. I just ate the food and didn't think much about it. But as I dove deeper into human health and nutrition, soil health became an important topic. It wasn't long before I was collecting my food scraps and taking them to the compost heap at the local community garden.

The health of a people can be no greater than the health of their soil. Soil provides nutrients to grow healthy plants, to be eaten by healthy animals, to be eaten by healthy humans. Soil that has been stripped of nutrients and polluted with toxins produces sick plants that are bland, tasteless, nutritionless, and even disease causing. In order to feed ourselves the best food, we must feed our soil the best as well.

In any wild ecosystem there is a synergy between plants and animals. Animals produce manure which decomposes into the soil. Plants die and litter the underbrush. From the death comes new life. Soil is enriched over time through the natural cycles. Topsoil accumulates. Soil becomes rich, black, and deliciously aromatic. Humus is created. In our more recent past, the link between animals and soil was vital. Grazing animals trample their poop into the grasslands, which grow back stronger. Various manures are spread into the soil to feed the diverse microbiome. Plants and animal bits are tossed into a compost heap, watered, turned, and reapplied into the land. The plants suck up the micronutrients and pass them up to us.

It wasn't so long ago that human poop was commonly composted as "night soil". It used to be standard courtesy as a dinner guest to give the host land some humanure in their compost toilet. In much of the developing world this is still true toay. But as populations grew denser and diseases become concentrated, humanure has become riskier as a source of disease and pollution. It's still possible to safely use our waste as fertilizer via composting, especially for trees and flowers. But our cleaner solution has been to totally disconnect our waste from the land entirely, which while limiting gross diseases, has broken an ancient chain between us and the soil.

The disconnect is even worse in wide spread animal agriculture. The majority of food growing doesn't even use compost or manure- just the spray of chemical fertilizers. The animal manure is instead collected in massive manure lagoons, which become a toxic environmental hazard because of the toxic food and chemicals the animals are given. The soil is deprived of millions of tons of waste that should be recyclable, and instead it pollutes our air and waterways. This fragmented system has too many external costs in degradation of our land, environment, and people to continue forever. We need another solution.

I'm not suggesting we return entirely to ancient methods. Our farming ancestors didn't always know what they were doing. The Sahara Desert was once fertile jungle, forest, and pasture before being destroyed by overgrazing, over farming, and dramatic shifts in weather. Babylon, the capital of the Fertile Crescent and the birthplace of agriculture is now dry abandoned ruins. Indigenous farmers burned forests for pasture and farmland, which enriched the soil in the short term but if poorly managed could give an edge to the desert. Sand, wind, and humans is a brutal combination of forces on any environment that can erode the lushest tropics into desolate wasteland in a short time. No, humans have been farming ignorantly since the beginning. We have to create a new solution for the future.

The answer may be in the rise of modern, science-based organic farming. Without the use of fertilizers, organic farmers have no choice but to use composts and manures to grow their crops. Even better are biodynamic farmers who keep animals to produce their own composts, dropping the manure transport chain to zero and integrating everything on their own farm. The proof is in the food. It's more vibrant, more beautiful, tastes better, is more nutritious, and is becoming higher in demand. The people are speaking through the market, and the health of the soil is gaining importance.

There's a lot of pleasure to returning our food scraps to the soil. More people are realizing that we shouldn't be tossing all our compostable waste to non-agricultural landfills and are collecting their waste for backyard worm bins, small gardens, and citywide composting programs. The health of the soil is a societal problem, and individual composting is a societal solution.

The Earth is alive. If you have any doubt, throw a handful of dirt under a microscope and you'll see a whole new world. It should be obvious that we need to keep the Earth alive to keep ourselves alive, but in many ways we seem hellbent on destroying the Earth and ourselves with it. Is it intentional self-destruction? I think it's a combination of ignorance and laziness and the onus falls on the educated and nourished to do something about it. And it starts with taking the scraps from your next meal and returning them to the soil.

Plants and Animals

Plants and animals go together like birds and trees, worms and dirt, flowers and bees. In every environment, every ecosystem, plants and animals depend on each other. Animals eat plants or eat animals who eat plants. Plants eat decomposed animal matter through the soil. It's a symbiotic relationship in nature, and they play well together in farming too.

The big concentrated system is unnatural in the separation of plants from animals and it causes problems. The soil suffers, the environment worsens, the plants don't grow as well, the animals get sick, and we don't get the best food from it. Our food system deserves an integrated solution.

Even if you want to focus on growing only organic plants for human consumption, animals are still your friend. First, they provide a trustworthy source of manure for your plants. Second, they make use of leftover scraps and unsold produce. Unwanted carrot tops, beat tops, turnip tops, and weeds make good food for sheep. Overripe fruit that didn't get out in time make good food for pigs. Just about anything extra makes good food for omnivorous chickens who love a high bug environment. This extra stuff could go to a compost heap, but it will do a better job of that if run through animals first.

You probably don't eat all the food you prepare or put on your plate, and that slop ought to go to chickens, pigs, or worms. We don't need millions of pounds of uneaten food going to landfills with manmade junk. This extra food should be going to our animal associates who will enrich the soil now and pay us back later in meat. It varies per animal, but in general for every five to ten pounds you feed livestock, it grows two pounds and produces one pound of meat. This doesn't sound that efficient except when you consider that food wasn't going to be eaten by anyone anyway. It's a way to make something out of nothing.

You might not have the space for very many animals, but even a worm bin on your window sill is valuable to growing better herbs and spices. It doesn't take much space to house backyard hens and it will be worth it for the eggs. If you have a lot of space for flocks and litters that's great, but if not you can still do plenty with a small system.

Plants and animals working together is the norm. We get higher productivity from the overlap. It's more complicated, but it's more natural. It works better. Together we make for happier plants, happier animals, happier soil, and happier people.

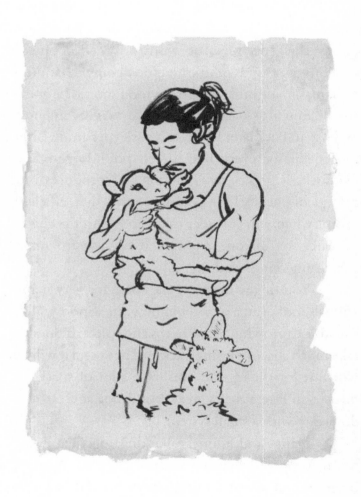

Grazing

For millions of years, countless giant grazing mammals roamed the world's grasslands, plains, prairies, savannas and bushes. Human hunter-gatherers often depended on these animals as a source of meat, tools, and clothing. About 10,000 years ago we domesticated the survivors, taming the aurochs into cattle, the mouflon into sheep, and the bezoar goat into modern goat. And we have continued to depend on them for meat, clothing, milk, and food security.

What's often overlooked in grazing animals is their role in soil building and carbon sequestration in stabilizing our environment. Grasslands produce as much or more vegetation as forests. Because of the shorter life cycles of grasses, they pulse carbon into the Earth faster than trees. Grasses are about half root, and as they are eaten and trampled, they shed these roots as carbon into the soil. As the herd moves on, the grasses regrow, and the cycle continues. This is the carbon pump. This is how the relationship between grazing animals and plants should work.

But over the last few hundred years the natural cycle has been broken. Land ownership has been cut into smaller and smaller chunks of human ownership. Wild grazers have gone extinct in many areas. Domestic grazers have been concentrated into small confinement cities, being fed indigestible corn, chicken manure, and animal bits instead of grass. The grass is left to grow into dangerous wildfire brush, the manure never makes it back into the soil, and the gas biproducts have nowhere to go but up into our environment. It's reasonable to be outraged, but don't be mad at the animals. The problem is clearly mismanagement by humans.

Grazing continues as it should in cases in the form of pasture farming. Electric fencing is a powerful modern tool to manage the animals and the land. Pastured beef goes for a premium, because it is tastier and healthier. The meat is packed with more nutritional punch. The animals aren't sick and cancerous, and those diseases won't be passed on to the eaters. The animals live as they should.

Critics will say that pastured grazing won't scale the same as concentrated systems. They overlook the true costs of that system- all the land required to grow the grains, all the energy required to transport the grains, the land destroyed by toxic manure biproducts, the damage to the environment, the sickness of our people. It might not scale to the same degree, but it doesn't have to, because our current way of doing things is leading us towards destruction.

Look to the buffalo. There were nearly as many animals grazing the Great Plains before settlers came as there are factory cattle in the USA today. It wasn't an environmental problem then. Grazers graze. It is the symbiotic nature of omnivores and plants, going back time immemorial. We have broken the connection between animals and land and there will be a price to pay. We will have no choice but to heal the link. Modern animal farming could destroy us, but if done right, it might just save us. The answer is in returning to pasture.

Death

I love these animals. I care for them. I feed them before I feed myself. I get up early on the weekends for them. I bring them grain, slop, and freshly cut grass. I take them on walks through the orchard. I maintain their housing and change their bedding. I weed and water their yards. I collect their precious poop and store it for later use. I give them medicine when they're sick. I swing by their house just to hang out with them. I call them by name and grow fond of their personalities and smells. I love them. How can I eat them?

How do you slaughter and eat your friend? How do you skin and cut them? How do you hang with someone every day of the year just to lead them out to pasture and kill them? With some remorse and regret. With the most gratitude, thanks, and appreciation. With love. Maybe a few tears shed over a burial ceremony on the land where we lived together. With friends, teammates, and family over a summer solstice celebration. In the cafe for lunch on a Wednesday. We do it together.

Death is a challenging topic of discussion when it comes to eating. Animals die for us, and so do plants. Evil "weeds" have their roots yanked from the ground. These carrots died for our sins. The salad leaves scream in pain through pheromones that alert their neighbors to bitter their leaves and toughen defenses in advance of threats. Food and death have a close relationship. How do you handle it? Do you eat some living things but not eat others? Do animals feel but plants don't? Where do you draw the line?

I care most about how that life form lived. Were the plants and animals happy? Did the animals frolic in the fields? Did the chickens express their chickenness picking bugs from the ground? Did the sheep express their sheepness in the pasture? Did the pigs express their pigness rooting in the ground? Did the fruit trees grow up root-sharing in a family? Did the greens get nutritious soil, sun, and water? Did the farmers do it with love?

I have a much easier time killing and eating my friend if I participated in his healthy, happy life than if he spent his time cramped in a factory with no room to move, tail chewed off by the animal behind him, chewing on the tail of the animal in front of him, pooping through slats, eyes, nose, and lungs stung with fecal matter, eating poisoned food, stomach lining breaking down, hoping for death. I want to know that the food was prepared with love every step of the way. I believe as death eaters, it is our responsibility to participate in life giving.

If we must die, we would all like to die with dignity. It should be quick and painless. Our loved ones holding our hands, a bright light in the distance. The reality is that it can at times be a long and drawn out struggle or a startling surprise. No one wants to die, but all of us must experience it. The best we can do for a dying community member is be there with our presence and love. To gather around our loved one, hold hands, and pray. To hold each other close and gather again over the next meal.

It would be nice to become food in the afterlife. To have our bodies buried beneath the trees, our ashes scattered in the fields. To enrich the soil and be reborn in the creatures that eat you. To crawl away with the bugs, carried off by the birds, sucked up by the trees. To live on in many things, literally, physically. I find it very comforting. The animals and plants will live on in us. And eventually, we all are eaten by the Earth. And maybe one day the Universe eats us all back.

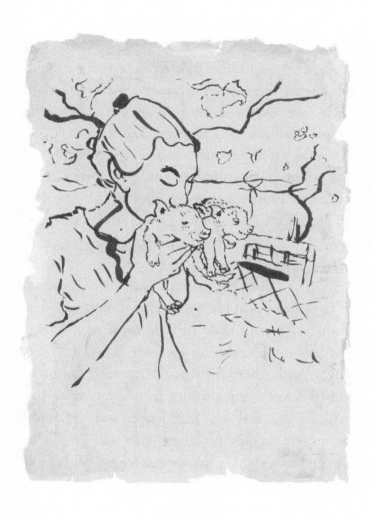

Caring for Animals

It is in our blood to love and care for animals. Humans are not solitary creatures. We prefer to live in extensive social communities, not just with other humans, but especially with animals. Our deepened relationship with animals, more than each other, is what allowed the progress of our society from subsistence hunter gathering to today. Dogs helped first with our our hunting, and then with our herding, of pigs, goats, sheep, cattle, chickens, turkeys, horses, llamas, alpacas, camels, and so on. Our society could not exist and our progress would not have been possible without working with these creatures. They provide us food security with their meat and milk, clothing in their skins, and crop fertility with their manure. There are important rational reasons for keeping them, but more than anything we feel an instinctive and emotional attachment to them. They give us joy. Their company feels right. They are our friends and family. We love them, and they love us.

When it comes to caring for animals, we can thank our ancestors for selectively breeding the friendliest, most responsive, and easiest to manage animals over the last 10,000 or so years. Every species is different, but the same fundamentals hold true to maintaining a harmonious relationship. My approach has three keys- responsibility, respect, and rewards.

It is a massive responsibility to be the caretaker of another life form. As a caretaker, it is your responsibility to show up every day. It is your responsibility to read, research, YouTube, visit nearby practitioners, and form mentor relationships. The Hawaiians have a word for responsibility and obligation called "kuleana". Once you kuleana, you can't un-kuleana. You are responsible from start to finish, so think seriously before taking responsibility.

Respect this animal. This is an intelligent life form that is smarter than us in its own unique way. It has a unique being, body, mind, behaviors, tendencies, desires, fears, likes and dislikes. It's being was shaped by wild evolution and our domestic history. Tai Lopez likes to quote Allan Nation as saying, "Don't try to teach a pig to fly. It can't do it and it bothers the pig". Respect the animal to know its nature. Don't try to force it from doing things that go against its being. Put it in an environment where it can naturally express itself. Dogs hunt, sheep graze, goats browse, pigs root, birds scratch and peck. Different animals want different bedding, different houses, different food, and different treatment.

Respect the animal to know what it wants and what it doesn't want.

Reward good behavior and punish bad behavior. Respect the animal to know what reward is appropriate. A dog doesn't want barley and a sheep doesn't want a bone. Be responsible to carry rewards on you when interacting with the animal. Try not to punish behavior that is natural to the animal. Goats climb and chickens don't roost until dusk. Don't force them. Preempt bad behavior by steering the animal towards another option and rewarding that first. Be persist and abundant in your rewards. Reward the animal for it's cooperation by giving it the best life you can.

It is becoming increasingly important to practice responsible meat production in a way that allows for happy animal lives while enriching the land and the environment. The industrial system is not good, but it won't fix itself. We need individuals to step up as stewards as our ancestors did. This work is one of the most challenging things you can do in terms of time, energy, and emotional difficulty of slaughtering and eating. But it is extremely rewarding in the daily joy, companionship, and gratitude to the life form. We've come this far together as a family, and we can't do it alone. We need to step up for them now more than ever.

Eating Animals

I tried vegetarianism and veganism for a while. Why support concentrated animal feeding operations that treat animals horribly and make people unhealthy? Do these creatures really need to suffer? Do I want to contribute to environmental damage? Could meat be bad for me? Could I be the one to kill the animal? Hard questions to answer. I felt the dilemma. I relate to people who want to abstain. I respect it. I tried it. But it wasn't for me.

The first thing I missed was the meat. I felt weaker and lower energy without it. I missed the taste. I missed eating it. But when I came back it wasn't for mass produced or fast food. It was for local duck eggs and pastured beef. I bicycled by these animals and saw them living decent lives outside. I spent more money for less food. I didn't have to support harmful systems. I could still vote with my food dollars. And I could be healthy doing it. I knew most of the health studies weren't controlling for quality of food, so it was a good bet to go for higher quality if I was going to be eating it. Humans are omnivores. We have plant teeth and we have meat teeth. So I started eating meat again.

When it comes to farming animals, a lot gets missed when people speculate and theorize. You learn what's real when you're out there on the land. Say for example, you're farming organic beets and carrots for human consumption. You're a produce farm trying to support alternative plant food for humans. But wild hogs start coming in from the back of the valley at night time and raiding your crop fields. You could go out of business if you let this continue. What do you do? Your job is to feed people, not pigs. You could try walling in all your acres, but pigs dig under. You could kill them, but a good middle ground is trapping them and raising them. It's better to try to give them a good life on the farm then to shoot them dead. You don't have unlimited options. You may eat them eventually, but that's not the point. You can send these pigs in to turn compost piles and clear out old root fields. But most importantly, you have their manure for the plants.

Plants need animals too. There isn't a natural ecosystem out there that doesn't have plants and animals living together. Even if you're eating plants, those plants probably ate animals- whether it was the manure, the bones, or the blood from the soil. If you care about growing good food, you have to take soil nutrition seriously. If you don't feed the soil you aren't going to have healthy plants. There are a lot of options to feed the soil, but there's no magic like recycling good old animal poop for compost. Where concentrated animal feed operations turn their poop into massive hazardous waste, small and medium farms turn it back into better plants. It's worth keeping animals just for this, and if you're keeping animals, occasionally there's situations where it's most respectful to eat one. I see so-called vegan farmers turn to flexitarians and eat meat at these times. At certain situations meat eating makes sense.

If all meat is from concentrated animal feeding operations, I say fine, don't eat it, you don't need it. But you can instead support your local farmers who are growing a better system. You can be healthy, you can support the environment, and you can contribute to healthier and happier animal lives. You can feel satisfied that your eating habits are making a difference.

When it comes to the final question of whether you can be the one to kill the animal, I'll tell you it's not easy. I've raised animals from babies, loved them, named them, connected with them, visited with them every single day, and been the one to lead them out to slaughter. Honestly, it can be traumatic. I have cried. I have missed them. It has changed the way I think about meat. But if anything, it has increased my appreciation and love for meat. I have greater gratitude for the animals. I don't want to waste any of the meat. I'm thankful for the sustenance, and I'm thankful for the animal to live on in me. It's not always easy to eat meat, but when the time comes, if done in the right way, I think it's the right thing to do.

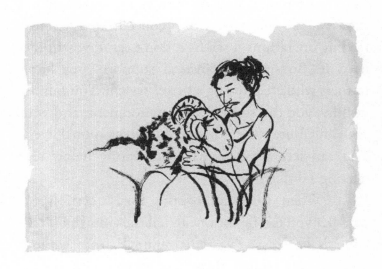

Hunting and Trapping

For two million years humans have been hunted for meat. Meat eaters eat meat. Sometimes they scavenge carcasses, but generally they hunt live prey. It is what it is. We could have domesticated animals sooner, but there was no need. There was such an abundance of massive wild grazers like the mastodon that it was simply a better strategy to hunt. Our transition from hunting to herding finally happened because of a shift in payoffs of the competing strategies. The evidence is in subcultures that were exposed to farming but switched back to hunting for hundreds more years until their ecosystem tilted to where farming became a necessity. Over time, the mastodon died out. The wild herds thinned. Hunting was no longer as productive. The cards shifted, and herding became the superior strategy.

But still, we hunt, fish, and trap. Not as a primary food strategy; it will never be again. Farming is here to stay. But we continue to hunt, not merely for sport, but to balance ecosystems and for supplementation of high-quality meat. Wild game is delicious. It generally lived a better life than its farmed counterparts. It moved more and ate a more varied diet. It might be a bit leaner and tougher, but it's usually healthier. So if we don't hunt, we seek it out. I look forward to wild game from Alaska or the local bush of Hawaii to add as a treat to my diet.

Of course, fishing has been a huge part of the equation. It's one reason why the vast majority of humans congregate around water. Commercial fishing continues large scale, but like hunting, possibly not for too much longer. Personally, I don't want my approach to fish to be "eat it until it's gone", but I do still want to enjoy it. I feel good about farming tilapia in our aquaponics system, growing taro root with nutritional help from the fish poop, and harvesting a couple times a year. It might not taste as good as fresh tuna, but it is sustainable and regenerative.

Situationally, hunting and trapping is necessary. Humans introduced wild goats that can destroy forest regions if left to multiply with no natural predators. Invasive fish can destroy an ancient reef ecosystem. A bear might find your trash can and learn to rely on it for food. Wild hogs might discover your beet fields and keep coming back as long as they live. While I've never shot a wild animal, I've trapped hogs when needed, clubbed fish, and eaten them. It would be nice if there was another way, but mother nature has a plan. Hunting will never make a major comeback, but it is a small piece of the puzzle, a component to The Food Life, and sometimes is still the right thing to do.

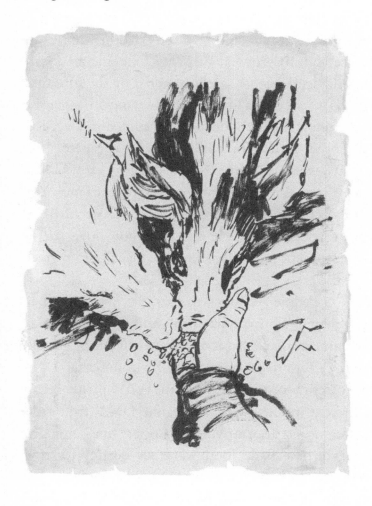

Growth

On one side of the fence, fruits and vegetables grow lush, vibrant, and easy. On the other side of the fence nothing grows at all. Why? One side randomly has shade, the other side is battered by the sun. One side is watered by a loving caretaker, the other gets no attention. One side is deliberately seeded and weeded, the other is left for wild weeds to compete. Like plants, we are products of our environment. Unlike plants, you can get up and move across the fence. You can weed and water your life. You choose where to plant your seeds. You can give more love to the environment around you, and you will grow green like the grass.

People are quick to blame genetics for their problems. We evolved from millions of years of winning humans. None of our ancient ancestors were obese. Our problems are more environmental. DNA may script our potential, but you will get vastly different results with the same DNA from two different situations. Modern society may not give you the best shade, food, water, or location to grow. You may be born on the wrong side of the fence. But you have some control over your environment.

Change your environment and you always have a fresh chance to grow.

Imagine growing food with and without love. If the farmers love the plants, animals, and soil, or if they don't give a shit and just need to make a few bucks. Loved soil receives compost, where unloved soil does not. Loved plants receive weekend weeding, unloved plants are sprayed with poisonous herbicides. Loved animals are walked, scratched, and treated, while unloved animals live under horrific nightmare conditions. What if a child receives love and attention, or isn't cared for at all? Love may be the biggest contributor to growth.

Young people should be encouraged to follow their love despite society's expectations. Social media tells you to look and act a certain way. Counselors tell you to get a stable secure job. Parents have your best interest at heart but are scared of you risking and failing. Imagine if more young people participated as loving custodians of their environment. If everyone weeded and watered their own garden, how clean and organized would our society would grow, how much better would our crops would grow, how much better would our food system would grow, how much healthier would our people would grow?

Trust

If you're going to trust anyone, you want to be able to trust the people who feed you. They are your life givers. You are in their hands. Hopefully they are feeding you good food grown with love, and not poison. You can't know for sure unless you investigate. You'll want to trust your farmer, and to do that you'll have to seek them out to know them personally. It's extra work, but it's worth it. Who knows where those chicken McNuggets came from? This question is leading more people to grow their own food or at least source it locally. If you go out there and look at how it's growing, you know whether you can trust or not trust the food.

Trust is in the food. How do you gain the trust of animals? If they're skittish, they might not let you feed them. At least until they observe you feeding a dog or cat in front of them. Then they come around your way. They observed your character and know they can trust you. Over time food can be used to train and gain trust of the most skittish animals. Feed enough animals consistently and you gain the trust of humans too. They see what you're about and will be happy for you to feed them too. If you mistreat animals and feed them food they aren't meant to eat, they will be sick, and they might not trust you. When people eat this food, they can become sick like those animals. If the animals don't trust their feeders, can you really trust eating them?

Uncle Ben told young Peter Parker, "With great power comes great responsibility" and if you choose to step into the role of a food grower, great responsibility comes with it. You have major influence in the health of the people you work with. You can heal them or make them sick. You owe it to them to work with integrity, and to be trustworthy. Be transparent. Invite everyone to check out your operation at any time. Let them show up and walk around. Let them know you trust them. Let them trust you.

Thank You Food

Thank you for this food. Thank you to the food. Thank you to the farmers for growing it. Thank you to the plants who gave their fruit. Thank you to the animals who gave their life. Thank you for our ten thousand taste buds to taste this. Thank you for the strength and nourishment I gain from eating this food. Thank you to God, to the Universe, for this next meal. Thank you. Amen!

Whether you are religious or not, there's something special about saying grace. Without it, you can get into a routine of taking the food you eat for granted. It's easy to forget about the farmers, the plants, the animals, the soil, the universe and everything else. A nice short reminder before the meal does so much for your life. A few words or a moment of silence is plenty to put you into the mindset of gratitude. The food tastes better and you get more out of it.

Gratitude is one of those things that gives you a lot more than you give it. Take two minutes to list all the things you are most grateful for. Try doing that first thing in the morning when you wake up. It sets a different tone for the day. It's hard to stay too mad when you have so much to be thankful for. Especially when you're thankful for the difficulties and challenges of life. Now try doing that before each meal and feel your hanger melt away. We realize that there's so much to be thankful for, just for the food, and life is good.

Food

Society

Eating to Save the World

Eating food is a political act. We are voting with our food dollars. Who do you support, organic integrity farmers or concentrated chemical farmers? Do you want a healthier and more secure society? Do you care about global warming and climate change? However you pay into the system you make a real impact. You influence the market and help economic sectors grow or shrink. You can say or even vote a certain way, but however your food dollars are going is how you really feel.

Yes, it is expensive to go all organic. And sometimes you want to support local restaurants that aren't sourcing organic ingredients. It's a challenge. But if you really believe in something, it sometimes means making a sacrifice. If you want to save the world it will take work. You may need to go out of your way, give up some, be picky, and spend extra. If you believe in it, go out and spend for it.

Sometimes you can affect the food environment by voting in the political system. Occasionally candidates care about it, or new policies have an effect. You do have a chance to make a difference. But a lot of the time it's just not relevant to the food system. It's not on the politician's radars. If you want to make a difference you can raise awareness on social media, but you have to put your money where your mouth is. Vote with your food.

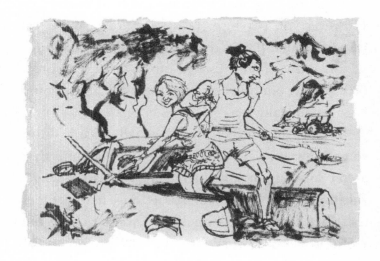

Food Freedom

Why can't I buy raw goat's milk without it being illegal? I should be able to buy apple chips made without a commercial apple chip processer. I should be able to buy meat that was slaughtered and processed where it was raised. I should be able to access pigs that were fed raw vegetable scraps from the kitchen without having the nutrients boiled out in a cauldron. Consenting adults should be able to legally buy the food they want from the source they want. I'm glad the government is trying to protect me from the grossness of concentrated animal feeding operations, but our food freedoms are being constricted in nonsensical ways. We should have more freedom to buy the foods we want to buy.

We can't legally sell our sheep or pig meat off farm unless it's processed at one of the few USDA approved abattoirs on the island. Restaurants would love to order it, but the government says "no, that's dangerous". The government wants to protect us from grotesque practices of industrial farming but at times the rules are oppressively restrictive on integrous operators. The impingements on our food freedoms are especially smothering to small and medium food businesses. A lot of things that would be nice and convenient are illegal, with only expensive and inconvenient legal alternatives.

There are possible solutions. One is under the table "farm sharing" as a semi-legal way to exchange the product. Jaywalking is illegal, but people do it anyways. Individuals can judge danger for themselves and choose. Broader scale we need some legal changes and that comes from personnel changes in our politics. Big Small Farmers doesn't have much lobbying power. We need politicians who understand food and can differentiate between the two-acre property that is selling one of their four goats and the nightmarish manure lagoon spewing robot-controlled cow city factory in middle America. These operations deserve different laws. In some cases there are distinctions, but in many important circumstances there aren't.

The answer many people are turning to for reclaiming their food freedom is growing it themselves. I can't legally buy raw milk? Then I'm going to keep livestock and do it myself. I can't buy meat that didn't go through one of the two legally certified abattoirs in my area? Then I'm going to raise my own hogs. I can't store unwashed eggs to increase shelf life? Then I'll eat them. Thankfully there aren't government controls over that. If anything, the government could liberate food eaters through small subsidies or even direct payments to citizens.

People are realizing that by handing over control of our most basic needs (to companies we don't really trust) we are also handing over some of life's greatest pleasures- feeding the animals, watching the plants grow, harvesting, washing, and eating our own home grown. By outsourcing all our food we're handing over our food freedom along with it.

I don't believe there is some specific government conspiracy to keep us from growing our own food. It was still being actively encouraged by the government into the mid-1900s with "Victory Garden" propaganda for post-World War II families. If anything there was a value change. Large farming became highly prioritized to feed the burgeoning worldwide boom in human population. Increased mechanization, scope, and scale were necessary. The idea was more machines means fewer farm laborers. The message was, "Get big or get out." Small farmers seen less as noble and more as dirty were free to escape to the city and do any number of cool professions. Somewhere in the noise people forgot how to grow and became wholly dependent on the big system.

If you have 100% trust in McDonalds and Monsanto to do the right thing, then keep doing what you're doing. If you put more trust in your local farmer, you can head on down to the co-op or market and vote with your food dollar there. But if you want a chance to fully reclaim your food freedom, maybe claiming responsibility and participating in the food system is the way to go.

Power

Remember when our leaders were participants in food growing and were experts in the food system? Our founding fathers may were farm practitioners with an understanding and interest of how to feed a society. Our early presidents knew that the health of a nation is tied to the health of the soil and they guided policy with that in mind. When's the last time we had an agriculturist for president? Times have changed. Nowadays our political leaders grew up in a different world far from the dirt, eating McFood ™ on their private flights. While our earlier leaders knew and cared about good food, our current charge doesn't seem to even have much awareness. It's not a partisan issue, it's a cultural dearth across the board.

Back in the day, our leaders and chiefs were the men and women of families who could reliably produce the most food for the tribe. These were often big, strong, people because they were best at securing the good food. In lean times you could trust and follow that they would lead you to greener pastures, abundant berries, and fertile hunting grounds. It was totally normal to follow the food leader.

But now, power over the food is concentrated in a few mega corporations who have corporate personage, a fiduciary obligation to be profitable to the stockholders, and massive lobby influence over the government. Size, scale, and scope are all that matters. Who cares about poison sprays, toxic runoff, manure lagoons, animal gas byproducts, melting ice caps, or positive cancer studies when the quarterly numbers are up? Meanwhile, our governmental leaders are like "sure, whatever" mostly because they just don't have the knowledge on the issue. It's not an evil system as much as it's neglectful. The machine has taken a life of its own and our society is educationally deprived of awareness, distracted by media scares, and too drugged off high-fructose corn syrup to act.

Imagine if our leaders came from organic farming backgrounds. Food knowledge would bloom. Policy would be shaped differently. The school system might actually educate people on food. Garden programs would be way more common. Subsidies might help smaller, organic farm businesses that care about climate, soil, and health. More families would garden. More young people would be incentivized to become farm entrepreneurs. Physical disease and mental illness would decline. Our world would become more vigorous and healthier, and farming would be a badass profession again. All possible in a world when farmers enter politics.

This isn't a job for me, or for most of us. I don't want to be Batman. But I would be sleeping a lot sounder and eating a lot better knowing that Batman is out there doing his thing. What I can do is raise awareness, campaign, and vote for Batman. I don't know who Batman is. They may be some organic farmer out there, with a successful business, understanding of the food system and social media, and a deep obligation to make a difference. I think if people saw this as a political option it would be a no brainer. A lot of people don't know it's important, but when they see it, they will intuitively understand.

It affects all of us. A third of Americans are obese and living with diabetes or prediabetes, and that number keeps going up. If it's not in our family, we have sick friends. We can sense that the food system has somehow failed us. The actionable solutions are not clear, other than personally growing good food ourselves. That's the route I'm going. But I'm hoping to have some farmers step up into politics, because if our leaders only gave a shit about our soil it could save us all.

Education

For millions of years, young people got their education on the land, helping with the food. They learned what plants were edible and which were poisonous. They learned how to trap and hunt. They gathered wood and cow chips for cooking fuel. They spent most of their time outside working and playing with the community. By the time they reached adulthood they had a strong practical knowledge, with useful skills, and were already contributing members of society.

Today's youth education is a different story. Young people are educated in schools. They go inside, sit still in rows, and are told to be quiet. If they can't, they're considered a problem, and may be given prescription drugs to sedate them. They are mostly asked to memorize and learn concepts that are helpful but aren't practical skills. They are strongly encouraged to go on to college, and if they do may be saddled with massive debt that severely limits their career and life options for decades. Few young people have any exposure to food education at all. When they graduate, they may still have no idea what they want to do and lack skills to contribute to society.

Consequently, our adults have no idea how food is grown, where their food comes from, and how their food affects them. The modern education system is broken, but rather than change the system we're trying to change the people. How do we fix the system instead? Maybe instead of college or even late high school, young people should have more choice to go to a trade school to learn practical schools, take agricultural work with afternoon classes, or work directly with mentors to build something.

The beauty of the switch from hunting and gathering to farming is allowing some people to be nonfarmers. Stockpiling of food allowed some people to pursue other sorts of work such as carpentry, blacksmithing, and so on. Now we have the need for all kinds of service work and a vast variety of jobs. Not everyone needs to be a farmer. Not everyone needs a food education. But is 1% of the population really enough to grow our food? Should 0% of our education really teach about agriculture in schools? This doesn't seem right.

Like most youth, I had zero exposure to food education from my schooling. There was no food or agriculture class. There was no school garden. We learned about plant photosynthesis and some chemistry, but never in respect to what we were eating. I had little idea how plants were grown and how the food system worked until I started self-educating later in my 20s. I never visited an organic farm until I was 25. If I had been exposed to agriculture much earlier, I probably would have pursued it. I was lucky to finally notice and become interested. How many would-be food growers never start because our food and education systems never bring it to their attention?

I'm optimistic about the future. I see school garden programs popping up everywhere. More school to farm tours. I see young people on social media discovering organic farming through beautiful pictures and choosing different routes in life. I see public leaders with real food knowledge sprouting up. I see more people learning agriculture through self-education and mentorship. I'm not sure if our education system will have a massive change to start prioritizing food knowledge, but I see more people taking education into their own hands, learning and teaching about food, and that's exactly what our society needs.

Exercise

You used to have to move to get food. For two million years we walked, hiked, ran, jumped, crouched, pounced, dragged, and carried to access the food we needed to survive. The past 10,000 has had more walking, squatting, bending over, lifting, carrying, lowering, swinging, chopping, and hammering. Either way you were living a very physical life, working in teams, walking 10+ miles a day, just to get your food and water.

Almost overnight McDonald's drive through came along and you don't even have to get out of the car. And now we have Uber Eats so you only need to move from the couch to the front door and back. From 10 miles to 10 minutes of walking a day. Welcome to the modern food lifestyle. Education and jobs have become totally disconnected from food. Most people sit at desks all day and come home to lie on the couch in the evening. It's a struggle just to get up from the couch to the bed at the end of the night. No wonder obesity and modern disease is still rising.

I always wanted to be a pro athlete. Not for the fame or money. Not because I had any pro athletes in the family. It was so that I could get up and move. I was the type of kid who couldn't sit still in class. It was way too boring. I fidgeted. I made sounds. Sometimes I got kicked out of class. I loved recess and PE. Fortunately, I dodged the Adderall over prescription epidemic. My normal hangout after school was either sports practice or the gym. I did pushups and pullups in the kitchen at night. I danced. I just loved to move any way I could.

When I succeeded in becoming a pro blogger with a 4-hour workweek I first structured my life so that it could be sports and exercise all the time. I spent two hours outside on the football field in the morning, three hours in the gym and on the basketball court in the afternoon, and 1 hour in the pool in the evening. I read textbooks on movement and body science. I felt healthy and good, but something important was missing still missing. A strong purpose. A clear impact to society. I could make content and share to help people move, think, and feel better, but maybe there was an even better way.

After I was introduced to farming it immediately made sense to me. It was athletic, physically challenging, and healthy. I was outside. I got to carry heavy things and walk long distances. I got to do a lot of different movements. It rewarded me for all that sports training and studying. But it also was for something very, very important and tangible. It was for good food that people would eat and have their lives changed. For a brighter future with healthy kids playing under fruit trees.

The more I farmed, the more I moved, the less I "exercised", the healthier I became. It has much less to do with genes than people think. It has more to do with environment and lifestyle. None of our ancient ancestors were obese. The healthiest people live physically active lives, but they don't necessarily exercise like we think of exercise. If you're using your body all day what extra exercise do you really need? Maybe a little stretch, swim, balancing yoga, and massage. An occasional heavy lift. It's optional. I was adopting the ancient lifestyle and feeling my best.

But if you're sitting or standing still for nine hours, how much can one hour of exercise really do? It can accomplish a little bit, but not enough to undo all the damage that comes with a sedentary lifestyle. Just like one organic salad can't undo a factory processed diet. You may have to change your lifestyle to change your life.

The question becomes, which jobs allow for you to best express your ancient humanness through movement? Which careers give you the potential for the best life, with the most built in exercise? I don't think it's an office lifestyle and I don't think it's pro athletics either. Having tried a few things, I would argue that it's organic farming. It has the most built in movement and brings you closest to the good food. After all, food collecting is our oldest work. It is the most comfortable and instinctual career. For many people it just feels right, if only they would get the chance.

When it comes to eating food, it tastes even better when you toiled in the soil for the plants and animals. The knowledge that your physical labor went into the meal makes it more delicious. You know it's more nutritious because you were loving at the very roots of this plant. It will make you feel better and give you more energy to get back out in the fields and keep on moving.

Farmville

For the first time, I found myself coming back every day to check on my crops and see how my animals were doing. Funny thing is, it wasn't real life- I was playing an online game called Farmville. The game came out in 2009 and within a year it had almost 100 million players. Huge numbers of people who had no farm experience whatsoever got a taste of the farm life through a Facebook app. If that ain't a sign of average people being secretly interested in agriculture, I don't know what is. I was one of those early Farmville players and it was one of my first influences towards The Food Life.

Games have been doing a better job of getting people interested in farming than our education system. I don't see 100 million kids in school gardens. Games are a different story though. Farmville is just one example. We've had Sim Farm, Harvest Moon, Agricola, Settlers of Catan, Minecraft and many more. Based on the popularity of these games it seems like access is the biggest obstacle between more people growing their own food. If people could drop their corporate and service jobs to manage a farm, I bet a lot would. Maybe they will if farm life blasts off again and urban farms come to a city block near you.

For me, at first, these were just games. I didn't think, "oh, I like farm games, so maybe I should be a farmer." The problem was I wasn't exposed to real life farms or farmers. The farm was just a fantasy setting like Hogwarts or Middle Earth. It was a cool alternate reality, but I didn't consider it a real thing. But when I finally started to come across farms it was like stepping into that fantasy realm. It was familiar. The ordinary things didn't matter in Farmville. Traffic, social media, and money were way less relevant. What mattered was the watering, the seeding, the weeding, the animals, the weather, the season, the food, and the farmers. I had played the game, and I found it even better in real life.

It's hard to say where games are going with immersive technology taking off on the horizon. People may plug their brains into a Matrix-style virtual reality while robots hold down base reality. Or maybe brain and optic implants for augmented reality will be the big trend. What's clear is that people will be going deeper into games with time. Games will become more realistic. Farm games will become more immersive, and you might even be able to virtually smell the soil. Things could go a couple of directions for society. I choose not to be scared. We should be optimistic. Gamers will come out of that virtual farm experience wanting more and seeing that as a real thing that they can experience. With technology taking over, the counterculture will more and more be the farm. The farm could be one of the few places where base reality is more immersive than virtual reality. Offices, apartments, and bland food will have no chance to match virtual reality, but the taste, smell, and texture of real-life Farmville has the best chance of prevailing.

Hefted

In James Rebanks' "The Shepherd's Life" he tells stories of an ancient shepherding lifestyle still practiced in some parts of the modern world. At the footsteps of the mountains of Northern England, when the grass grows rich in the summertime, all the shepherds in the community release their sheep to graze in the upper fells. Months later, before the weather turns to winter, they work in coordination with dogs to bring their sheep home. The sheep are unwatched for the season, the shepherds know they will still be there. Over time they have become hefted to that particular plot of land. It is their home and they won't stray far.

To be hefted is to be attached to home. It is a feeling of comfort associated with a place and the behaviors that return us to this place. To be hefted is to return home after a long day or a trip abroad. It is why dogs lost far from home return to find their owners. It is why we may move states, but still snack on the same comfort foods and look forward to returning home for the holidays. It is not just sheep that become hefted, but humans as well.

We don't like major change very much, even when they are good for us. We protest, we resist, we hang on to the old ways of doing things. It's human nature. Over time we become more and more stuck in our ways, attached in our behaviors, hefted to home. We are willing to make small changes, but only big changes under massive force.

The biggest obstacle to major changes in society- moves towards The Food Life- is that we are hefted to our current way of life. We may complain about the desk job, the traffic, the overuse of technology, the fast food, but if it feels like home, that's how we will continue to do it. Minor incentives aren't enough, and force of nature may come too late.

The hope for change is in our youth- bright eyed youngsters in their early 20s straight out of college who want to see and experience the world. They're attached to home but aren't likely to come back and live permanently with their parents again. They haven't yet established a new home or way of life. Their next experiences make a tremendous difference for their permanent future. They can only root and unroot so many times. So if they leave to go WWOOF, volunteer farm, and start growing something, that's the best chance that new farmers will stick. Ten years later they will be too hefted to change, but if they've embraced The Food Life by then they'll do it for a lifetime.

The shepherd's in James Rebanks' stories are hefted through the generations. Their great, great, ancestors were shepherds too. They have no desire to change. That's just how they do things. It says on the back cover that "Most stories are of those trying desperately hard to escape. This is a story of someone trying desperately hard to stay". If we aren't careful, it could all slip through our fingers and find ourselves back into the city chasing a paycheck. But even then, our attachment to the land can't be fully lost in a few generations- it goes back through the eons. We are hefted through blood. In a way we will always be attached to the land. So even if people are too attached to their status quo to make major changes, they might make the small changes of visiting their farmers and growing a little food in their back garden. That might be enough.

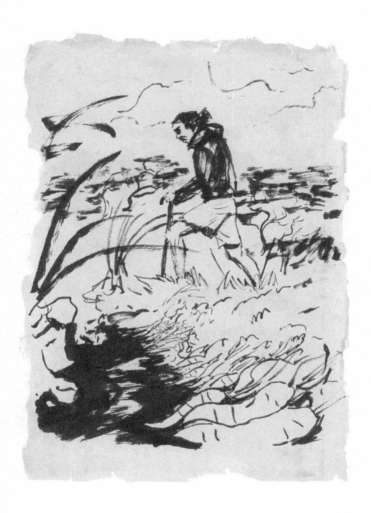

Eating

Food

With Bread

Companions- your best friend, your partner, your closest mate. Simply put, the people you spend the most time with. Companion comes from the Latin word "companis", "com" (with) + "panis" (bread). Companion's literal meaning comes from "with bread". Companions are who you eat with. And possibly who you work and grow grain with. The Food Life makes the best mates and it goes beyond eating. It goes into the working. When we toil and sweat together, we stay together to reap the rewards together. Farming is a team sport, and eating is a team celebration. It's better done with companions.

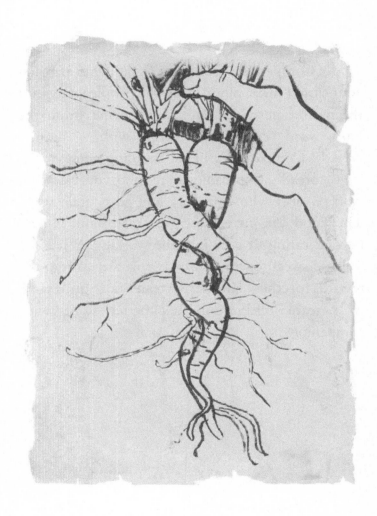

Food and Health

Modern society offers a lot of cool luxuries like the internet, fast transportation, a nearly unlimited food supply, powerful medicine, and so much more. But it also brings a host of modern diseases and illnesses- obesity, diabetes, cancer, autoimmune disorders, developmental problems, mental health, chronic depression, stress, and on and on. We live longer on average now than our ancient ancestors, but we're also sicker for longer and in more ways. What's the deal?

Modern sickness is caused by a lot of things. But most of those things have to do with modern lifestyle being a drastic departure from ancient lifestyle and biology. We're supposed to be walking 12 miles a day which circulates our fluids, not sitting in a chair for 12 hours. We're supposed to be soaking up vitamin D, listening to birdsong, with dirt between our toes, but now we're stuck in traffic, breathing in exhaust fumes, and distracted by noise pollution. We're supposed to be eating a wide variety of naturally colorful micro-nutrient rich foods to protect us from disease, not a narrow diet of highly processed corn and corn-fed meat.

Modern healthcare is great in a lot of ways, but severely lacking in others. Vaccines really do eradicate disease but it's hard to blame a parent for being apprehensive about shooting their baby up with 12 booster shots at one time. Antibiotics work great mostly, except when they create resistant superbugs and wreck healthy gut bacteria. There's not a lot of funding for studying food healing because you can't copyright a plant that grows in everyone's backyard. I recently received prescription produce vouchers as payment at the farmer's market, and while that gives me hope, it's new and rare. I don't see a lot of doctors prescribing vegetables because it's not commercially viable and it's the fiduciary obligation of these corporations to make money for their shareholders. The bottom line is, while modern medicine saves lives, there's so much more we can do as individuals to keep ourselves healthy.

You hear these crazy stories of people changing their diet and being cured of chronic illness, sometimes even cancer. It might not work every time, but I don't need to see a study to know that a fresh home-grown herbal tea is going to be better for my health than a high fructose corn syrup soda cocktail. It's on us as individuals to clean up our diets, and then we will have a healthier society.

Is it crackpot snake oil witchcraft to suggest that switching from a cubicle to a garden will improve health and happiness? It's no wonder so many young people are fleeing corporate culture and student loans for organic farming and animal caretaking while they can. It just feels right. It feels good. It feels healthy. And if it feels healthy, it probably is healthy.

Is it possible that we can cure illnesses of the modern world with lifestyle changes? Maybe, but it will take a lot of people and a lot of small things. You can't just push one button and it all changes. Not everyone can be a biodynamic organic farmer. We need those office workers, but they deserve a plant filled atrium to enjoy their walking lunch breaks. The centralized food system is great at feeding everyone, but we need some higher quality food options in the cities. We need more doctors prescribing plants. We need more politicians with farming backgrounds. We need more young organic food workers to spread their message through social media. I see no reason why we can't have all the good of the modern world with the health and happiness of our ancestors too. Let's start with a good choice on our next meal.

The Good Food Diet

You hear a lot of weird diet advice these days. Sugar is bad, so don't eat fruit. Gluten is bad. so don't eat bread. Carbs are bad. so don't eat greens or grains. Fat is bad. so don't eat cheese. Dairy is just freaky, so don't eat any of that. But protein is okay, so eat meat only. Actually, meat is really bad for you, only eat processed soy products. What? Something's not right here.

Could quality be the real problem? Maybe highly herbicided, pesticided, and chemically processed high fructose corn syrup is to blame, not blueberries and bananas. Maybe that gluten sensitivity is really glyphosate sensitivity. Maybe chronically stressed hormonally imbalanced cows aren't going to make the healthiest milk or meat. That translucent ice berg lettuce won't have the same nutrition as a dark leaf salad green. A factory chicken is not the same as a pastured chicken. Quality matters. What ever happened to a diet where you just try to eat good food?

A lot of people don't want to hear this advice because they don't want to spend more money, energy, and time on food. Food is expensive enough already, how can you afford to spend more on it? Good question, but here's a better one- how can you afford not to? You get what you pay for. You are what you eat. Cheap food makes a cheap body. A cheap body fuels a cheap brain and neither performs well. The expense comes later in low energy, poor production, poor health, medical costs, and shorter life. Personally, if I can at all afford it, I would like to pay more for food, not less, and I will gladly sacrifice to do so.

If you want to eat your healthiest, you must also care about how the soil was treated, how the food grew, how the animal was raised, how the food was processed, how it was shipped, and who were the parties involved. If you go with the low-quality option, no matter the configuration of macros, you're going to get lower quality results. But if you go with the higher quality option, you have a lot more flexibility in what you're eating and you're still going to get good results, because at the end of the day, you're eating a good food diet. It's not that complicated.

The biggest issue is usually access. Good food is expensive, but even if you have the money, it might not come to your area. You may live in a food desert. There may be no organic farms in a 100-mile radius from where you live. If that's the case, you're at a decision point. You've already taken the red pill and it will be hard to go back to eating what you've always eaten. But does that mean you have to leave for greener pastures? Possibly so, or it could mean growing it yourself. That's the solution we're seeing for more and more urban dwellers. You might not be able to grow it all, but some summer tomatoes and fall brassicas do make a dent in the diet. The good food diet is simple, but that doesn't make it easy. But few things that are worth it come easily.

Milk

When's the last time you milked a cow? While I had never milked an animal, I drank a lot of milk when I was young. Calcium is good and I wanted to grow strong bones. I was influenced by my favorite athletes in the "Got Milk?" campaigns, and my family was swayed by the USDA dietary guidelines that put dairy as an essential part of a daily diet. So my mom went to the supermarket and picked up milk that came from who-knows-where. Never mind that my Chinese father was lactose intolerant. I had plenty of stomach problems, but I ignored them and just kept on drinking milk. As I got older, I got skeptical. Is milk really that good for you, or is it a freaky and unnatural source of disease that is pushed by creepy Big Dairy? It's a complicated answer that depends on who you are and what you're drinking.

Human babies drink human milk, and it wasn't until about 10,000 years ago that we started drinking animal milk. Domestic herds gave us food security, especially in the winter. When the ground is frozen, and no crops will grow, animals give us our sustenance through meat, blood, milk, and warmth. Interestingly, while most farm crops spread rapidly from west to east along similar growing climates, herd

153

animals spread especially to northerly to areas with the harshest winters. Societies closer to the equator with longer growing seasons would welcome farm animals, but they could depend on year-round growing season for their food. Northerners would rely more on animals for better food security and extended living range during the winters. Thus, Northern European mountain goat people, Mongolian herders, and other wintery animal cultures who lived and worked closely with domestic animals.

Dairy culture wasn't just a diet, it was a lifestyle. These people cared for their herds- they sheltered, protected, and fed them in the winter time. They moved with them to pasture and guarded them during the summer time. They trimmed their hooves, gave them medicine, made clothes from their fur and skins, and of course milked them. The herders and herds lived a symbiotic lifestyle depending on love and respect for each other. Descendants of these people may be surprised to discover an affinity for grazing animals that comes from a mysterious place- it's in our blood.

Over the past 10,000 years, it was Northerners, especially Europeans, who drank the most animal milk. While not millennia, 400 or so generations was enough time for lactose digesting genes to spread rapidly across milk cultures. Those who could not digest it would be heavily disadvantaged. Most who survived acquired it. But many farming cultures continued without animal milk, and only began with the recent modernization of the food system- hence lactose intolerance across much of Asia, Africa, and indigenous America. Not everyone has the genes for it yet.

Over those 10,000 years of milking animals, herders kept a variety of animals. Goats were popular for their mobility in mountainous regions and ability to clear brush. Sheep were popular for their wool production in colder climates. Horses were popular for their agile transit. Cattle, while useful for dragging heavy plows, were nowhere near the dominant representation of dairy like it is today. In the modern industrial food system, cows are the largest dairy animal that produce the most milk. They scale the best. Under modern consumer scale dairy farming in America, cows represent almost 100% of all milk, while historically certain populations favored goats, sheep, or other sources for dairy. Consequently, cow milk might not be as digestible compared to goat milk to many people. But it's scale that matters to the big dairy companies.

Herd animals naturally turn grass and shrubs into milk through their special rumen stomachs. But in the industrial food system cows are forced to turn corn, other animals, and even sometimes chicken manure into milk. To produce more milk they are injected with hormones. To slow the deterioration of their stomach lining and other health problems they are injected with vaccines and antibiotics. All these unnatural processes are passed into the milk, which is passed on to us, which is manifested in "lactose intolerance" and other disease.

So is it good or bad to drink milk? It really depends. It depends on your family history. It depends on your genetics. It depends on what kind of animal the milk came from. It depends on what the animal was eating and how the animal was living. It's not an easy answer. It's up to you to research and depends on what you find.

My solution is to keep animals myself. I'm over the big dairy industry, but I'm drawn particularly to sheep. I know the Northern European side of my family depended on these animals for thousands of years. Unfortunately, their milk is not accessible in the large market, and even local raw milk is technically illegal to buy. It's hard to get. But we grow our herd, and coffee creamer in the mornings is more than enough. When it comes to drinking milk, my personal philosophy is, it's best to be close to the animal who produces it.

Fasting

As much as I love eating, I also love not eating. Fasting feels incredible. And when you look forward to that next meal for extra hours, it tastes even better. You may have heard about intermittent fasting or fasting windows. Basically, the idea is if you go longer between your dinner and your breakfast, you get better performance . If you eat the same food in fewer hours in the day, you will have better results. There's some truth to this, some history to this, and it feels great too.

Back in the hunting and gathering days, there was almost no storage of food. There was occasionally some fermentation going on, but people lived with only what they could carry. Farmers and herders could functionally store food in their grains and flocks, but even when salt became more common you couldn't stockpile in the way we do today. Salt lets you preserve more kinds of food for longer, and for thousands of years it was the main way to keep food. Now we have canning, fridges, freezers, and freaky foods that last forever on a shelf. But back in the day you probably were eating hand to mouth, day to day. If you're a man going out on the hunt, you might not eat anything until dinner time. You might not break fast for 20 hours since the night before. And you probably felt sharp with heightened senses because of being in that fasted "hunt mode."

The reason why your performance is better in a fasted state is because the head brain and the gut brain are in sort of a zero-sum competition for resources. The head brain has the most blood to think when your stomach is empty and inactive. Your gut brain is most efficient at digestion when your head brain is off. This is why you get so sleepy after eating a big meal, and why you have extra energy when you haven't eaten in a while. You can ruin your productivity and digestion by eating at the wrong time, or you can boost your productivity by extending your fasted state. It's good to either keep it in hunt mode or go for the full rest and digest.

We all have an eating window. Maybe you finish eating dinner by 7:30, don't snack, and don't start eating again until 8:30 in the morning. This would give you a 13 hour fast and an 11-hour eating window. I've tried 15 hours or more and have some friends who do the full 22 hours fast and two hours of eating. The longer the fast, the longer you can work at peak brain performance. Results vary, but I know that if you want to make yourself sleepy you should eat a big meal, and if you want to get some serious work done, you should start in the morning and push back your meal.

There's something about working on food while fasted that makes the food taste even better when it's time to eat. I love to feed the animals in the morning and feed myself later. If you're a parent you may be feeding the kiddos first, and that feels great for a lot of reasons.

You don't need to eat all the time. You may benefit from fasting more, without necessarily eating less. It will feel good physically. It will help you mentally. It will give you more appreciation for food and understanding for those who are struggling to feed themselves. And the longer you wait, the better that next meal will taste.

Slow Food

It's taken thousands of years of breeding to domesticate our modern varieties of edible plants and animals. It can take five years for a tree to produce fruit, one year for an animal to be ready for slaughter, three months from seed to carrot harvest, weeks to ship, dozens of hours of weeding, and a half day of cooking. Yet we want our food to be ready in five minutes.

Fast food has revolutionized food culture. McDonalds is everywhere. So many meals are eaten in cars. Expectations have changed and patience is thin. People want to eat right away, at the sacrifice of everything else. Forget nutrition, forget taste, forget freshness, I want it now! Historically, it's not normal, but in the modern age of rush hour traffic you can't really blame people.

It used to be that you could only eat what food was in season. You had to wait all year. You get Asparagus in the spring, tomatoes in the summer, potatoes in the fall, and oranges in the winter. But thanks to tropical growing and mass distribution you can get almost anything, anytime, anywhere. No wonder so many people don't cook anymore, let alone grow their own backyard produce.

Slow food is not about slow service. It's not about being anti progress. It's about not sacrificing quality in order to eat as quickly as possible. Good food simply takes longer. It takes longer to farm and longer to cook. You might not get it year-round because it doesn't ship as well. You're going to have to wait longer, but anticipation enhances the taste, and when it finally gets to your mouth, it will be that much more delicious.

Farm to Table

The only thing better than farm to table food is plant to mouth. Pulling a big juicy carrot out of the soil, wiping it on your dirty shorts and crunching into it right then and there. Snagging a ripe mango from the tree with your fruit picker and sticking up your face on the spot. Trapping a wild hog on your own land and fire roasting it for a hosted potluck. Harvesting salad in the morning and eating it for lunch. It does not get fresher nor better than this.

The beauty of local food is in the flavor and nutrition. Most foods are ticking time bombs until their expiration date. After peak freshness it's all downhill from there. Every mile traveled means more nutrients leached and more taste gone. The shorter the distance, the better. The closer proximity, the more we can focus on taste and nutrition rather than shelf life. It doesn't matter if it goes bad in three days if you get it on the first day. And it's going to taste oh so much better straight from the ground.

Shipping food long distance on a grand scale is a waste of fuel that might also be destroying the climate of our Earth. It also leads to tasteless and nutritionless food. Just look at iceberg lettuce. Does anyone LOVE iceberg lettuce? If not, then why are we doing this? Because it lasts on a shelf. It can sit in a container and stay at mediocre instead of going from good to bad. When you're shipping food out, these things matter.

I'm all for eating exotic and rare foods from around the world. I'm very grateful to be able to eat out of season fruits and vegetables shipped in from winter growing in California. I don't think you're a bad person for eating food that used fuel to get to you. But I do recommend trying out some local fresh food, just for that extra taste. Your best bet are the greens and fruits. If you didn't think you liked your vegetables, you may be surprised by what a short travel distance can do for taste and texture. If you can get fresh local meat, it's game over- there may be no going back.

You'll have to go out of your way to get fresh food, because it's not fresh for long. You'll have a chance to snag it fresh from the ground at a farmer's market. If you're lucky there might be a nice co-op store in your town. Maybe there's some trendy restaurants that source local food and even have an herb garden in the back. Or you could take the leap and start growing wherever you are right now. Even a small square plot can make for some nice greens, or a few summer tomatoes to pop in your mouth.

There's nothing quite like that crunch, especially when it came from your own backyard.

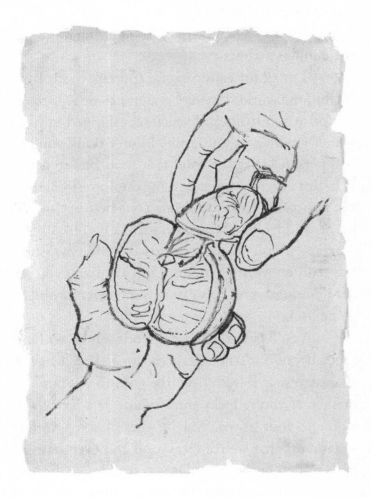

God in the Food

You can't tell me God isn't in this mango. Why is it so juicy? How is it so sweet? Why does it taste so good? Why do we have 10,000 regenerative taste buds to experience this food? Is all that purely chance? You could choose to believe that. I think it's God. And God must love us, because it doesn't have to taste so good, but it does. God is in the food, I believe it.

It's not something rational that can be proven. Some would argue it can be disproven. But it makes sense when you bite into that perfect meal. Why not take a moment to give thanks to the universe and Earth for providing us this sweet sensory meal? Does it hurt to believe that God loves us through the food?

I wasn't particularly religious as a boy. My parents didn't talk about it too much. A lot of my smart friends were atheists and agnostics. Seattle wasn't the most religious place, but we did go as a family to a Unitarian Universalist Church and I was exposed to a variety of religious beliefs and religious communities. I held the Bible, the Quran, the

Bhagavad Ghita, and the Tao Te Ching. As I grew I became more aware.

For a long while I cared most about what was provable, true, and rational. If it couldn't be proven, it was fake and only a fool would believe in it. But as I learned more, I realized how little I knew. Where does gravity come from? Where do the rules of the universe come from? Why are things the way they are? There are things we will never know, but we can know this- the universe is a vast place with power we will never fully comprehend. God is in the perpetual mystery, the unknown, the powers behind the powers.

I began to care less about what was certain, and instead care more about what was useful. I wasn't certain that God loved me, but it seemed like a useful thing to believe, so I started going with it. I began looking for God's love in everything and saw it wherever I looked- in the sun, in the stars, in the moon, in the ocean, in the soil, in the plants, the animals, and especially in the food. And if God is in the food, of course God is in everything.

I used to have a lot more confusion over life and fear of death. But as I became more trusting in the love of God, I felt more certainty over life and comfort in death. Life itself is a manifestation of God's love, and death is simply a return. God brings us into this world and holds our hand as we go back to the universe. Faith gave me strength.

What a blessing of love from God in the pleasures that we feel from our environment, especially eating. It doesn't have to taste so good, but it does. It doesn't have to feel so good, but it does. I wish that blessing upon the plants who eat the sun on their skin and drink the water in their roots. I wish that blessing upon the animals who eat the grass. I wish the blessing of God's love on all things as they feed and become food. I may not be able to prove that it's real but believing makes life a lot richer. So thank you God for this.

Growing Food

Automatic Farming

At first there was man with stick and woman with seed. Together they prayed for rain. When this was good they ate and had children, so there were more humans. Then the man began to drag a plow and the woman carried buckets of water, while his son and daughter removed weeds. A beast began to drag the plow, carry the water, and eat the weeds, so there were more beasts. Humans now had much more free time to do everything else, so they built civilization, and machines. Then a machine began to drag the plow, so there were more machines. The machines began to dig, haul, harvest, and drive the humans. The beasts lost their jobs but were kept for milk and meat. Oxen were displaced by tractors, horses were replaced by automobiles, and new combine technology sent humans into to the cities to work on more machines.

Automation advances around farming allowed humans to farm larger areas with fewer people. Now a single person on one tractor could do all the ripping, tilling, planting, spraying, and harvesting that previously took hundreds of laborers. The proportion of farmers dropped from 90% to 2%.

This new system wasn't the most efficient in terms of yield per acre or quality of yield, but it was the most efficient in terms of yield per labor, and it scaled easily enough to feed the burgeoning masses. So people took jobs elsewhere. But now many of those jobs are becoming subject to automation too.

Warehouse robots have replaced human manufacturing jobs, self-service checkout stands have replaced cashiers, AI voice robots have replaced call center workers, online apps are replacing accountants and lawyers, truck drivers will soon be replaced by self-driving vehicles, and on and on. We're entering a future where fewer humans do work of any kind, because it's hard to compete with autohumans that don't eat, sleep, or need to be paid. The jobless masses are turning to drugs, suicide, and immersive alternate realities, but I think given the option most of them would like to do some kind of work if they could. So what will they do?

One area where human labor is still very welcome is in intensive organic farming. We've automated food growing to scale, but we're unlikely to automate to depth as well as humans can do it. A tractor is great at turning and spraying large acreage, but small human hands stay great for weeding perennial plants. A system for automatic farming monocrops is simple enough, but a small biodiverse garden with vertical stacking has the complexity that requires creative human minds. The next step in improving our food system is a more labor, and the next step for society is liberation of laborers, so more people growing food seems like the likely inevitable.

There's a question of how the jobless masses will be able to afford to live. Growing some of their own food is certainly part of the answer. Perhaps a universal basic income will arrive soon, taking labor profits from big technology companies and paying back the workers who were replaced. Our machinated future doesn't have to be dystopian. There is an opportunity to reenter the garden. The wealth created from mass automation could be redistributed throughout society, ushering in a new prosperous era with increased standard of living for the common people. They can take their tech funded check, grow their own food, and live better lives.

In the not so distant future we may see a surge of new food growers. Cityscapes will turn into urban forests with rooftop gardens. Fruit orchards will grow out of parks. Abandoned lots will be claimed as community gardens. Every man, woman, and child will have a small worm bin on their porch. As robots automate many of the non-food jobs, humans can get back to our oldest tradition, what we do best, growing and eating food.

How to Start Farming

As I tell my story I have more and more people ask me how to start farming. Their stories are often like mine and my friends. Maybe you're sick of your corporate job and want something healthier and more meaningful. Maybe you've been lucky enough to travel the world and see farming as a good way to settle down. Or maybe you feel a strong urge to start growing and want to farm because it feels just right. Whatever your reason is, I can advise future farmers based on my own experience.

The farm industry has evolved through new technology, but in some ways it's frozen in the past. Getting a farm job usually doesn't work like getting a white-collar job. You might need a resume, but probably not. You need to prove yourself first instead. Usually the route to professional farming goes from part-time volunteer to full-time volunteer, to intern / apprentice, to professional. You should expect to be paid only in food in the beginning. Eventually you will be paid money. You must be patient. The crops don't grow overnight. They take seasons.

For me, I just started showing up to the closest volunteer day to where I lived. It was a small community garden. I enjoyed it, was learning, and it fulfilled me in the way I hoped, so I kept going. From there, some other regular volunteers invited me to a volunteer day at a larger farm nearby. They didn't invite me the first time they met me though. It wasn't until they saw I kept coming back. So I started going to their Friday volunteer day, and eventually their Wednesday volunteer day. After a while I could have become a more dedicated intern, then an employee, but instead I moved and took the same path at a different farm in Hawaii. First, I volunteered part time, then full time, then finally signed a paid contract.

The best way to start is to go to the nearest volunteer day and start there. If you're lucky you will be referred to it, but you may need to search it out. Ask friends, use social media, keep your eye out for gardens and farms that you may pass in your daily travels. Show up and see if you like it. If you don't like it, you saved yourself a lot of time. If you do like it, keep showing up, be eager to learn, keep your ears open for opportunities, and trust that in time you will be a pro.

I advise you to not try to do it yourself at the beginning. Get some hands-on experience as a volunteer learning with practicing mentors and teachers. If you try to launch it yourself, you are much more likely to fail and burn yourself out. Later once you have learned successful models and techniques you can start something up if you like. But if you want to continue to work on other's land and projects there's no shame in that either. Not everyone can be in charge. You'll get your turn later if you want it.

When it comes to getting land, it's a lot easier than you would think. You don't necessarily need to put up the cash to buy some expensive farm land. There's lots of old, neglected farms out there that have failed to pass hands in the generation because of people leaving the farm, or death and estate taxes. In many cases landowners will gladly lease land to a grower either for cheap or even for free, just to have the land productive again. Remember, when you're farming the regenerative way, you're improving the value of the land and providing a service for the landholder. They could even pay you for that. There are plenty of other ways too. You can get plots in community gardens, university sponsored programs, or government programs. Keep on the lookout for farm lease deals, because they are out there. You may not have the peace of owning the land, but you won't have the stress either, and you will be able to treat it like your own.

When it comes to doing anything you want to do, the best bet is to get started as soon as you can. You don't want to wait, looking out the window wondering what if you got started earlier. If it's something you want, try for it today, not tomorrow. Don't quit your day job just yet. Try it out during your free time, and if it's right for you, you'll naturally grow into it over the seasons.

Accessing Land

A lot of people want a plot of land to grow food, keep animals, and live with friends and family. But we keep making more people and they aren't making any more land. There's a supply / demand problem and no wonder real estate and housing keeps climbing in price. A lot of people want a plot of land, but a lot of people can't have a plot of land. It's a dream not everyone can achieve. Or so they say. The truth is it seems to be a lot easier than most people think.

First, you have at least your front porch, and you might have a backyard and roof access too. You don't have to wait until you have money to buy property to start enjoying the pleasures of growing and harvesting your own food. I have friends who grow rosemary, basil, and other herbs on their porch in the city. It's not a huge commitment but they get a lot out of flavoring their dinners. I have other friends who are growing edible microgreens in their basement under UV lights. Land access is not a real problem to getting started. If you want to scale larger, there's plenty of opportunity for that too.

There's a lot of neglected agricultural land out there owned by old people with no young farmers to take it over or that was inherited by young people who have no desire to farm. Some people want The Food Life, but a lot of people are tunnel-visioned in the city bubble and don't. Right now there is more demand for young growers than there are young growers. If you network with the right people you can access land easily.

The easiest way to start is jumping on someone else's land. There's plenty of community garden plots out there for free or low lease. There are programs to hook you up. You can start growing on someone else's land and take ownership. It becomes yours, not in the legal way, but in the sense that you are the caretaker and guardian of this land. We have beekeepers who manage hives on our lands, and all they give in return is a little honey and the gift of bee pollination. I took over several pasture areas to manage for livestock. A girl claimed rows and beds for growing flowers to sell on the side. Another farmer moved their personal chicken flock up to the farm. Our names aren't on the title deeds, but it doesn't matter. Even our farm manager doesn't have legal ownership, but he takes personal ownership.

As you grow your roots deeper into the community you will access more and more land opportunities. You might be able to jump on a big plot of land, and as long as you are fixing it up, cost doesn't have to be a problem. Remember, if you are raising the value of their land, you are doing them a service, and you may even be paid for the service of farming someone else's land, as well as reaping the rewards of the harvest. You may not have as much legal security in your time investment, but with good relationships it's as good as yours.

Private property is a relatively new concept, an invention forced by increasing populations on the same area of land. Before, communal land and farming was much more normal. Why would you want to separate yourself and do your own thing anyways? Ancient humans knew that teamwork makes the dream work and did it together. If you helped grow it, you would also be there to reap the rewards. You had security in community, and while times have changed the same principles hold true.

Don't wait until you can save up the money to buy land and start farming. Don't be discouraged by how daunting that looks, because there's an easier way. If you want to get working on the land, just get started with what lays around you, and with the right work and partnerships, in time it will become yours.

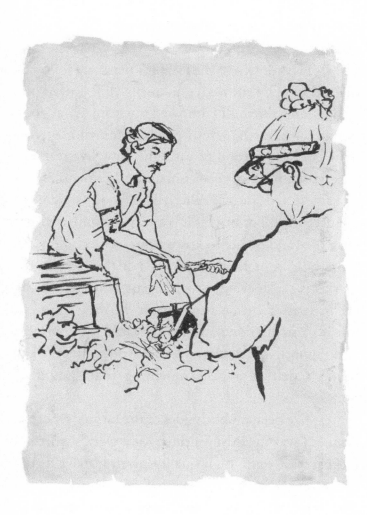

Markets

I was drawn to the farmer's market. I followed the crowds, I followed the smells, I followed the sounds, and above all I followed my stomach. A good farmer's market has fresh produce for your weekly haul, good fresh food to eat right now, live music, a grass patch for you to sit on, and other people who are interested in the alternative food system to connect with. For buyers it is a way to connect closer with the food, to get to know your farmer, and learn more how your food is grown. For the farmers the market is a sales event, a social event, and a marketing event. It isn't always necessary to run the business, but it's usually done anyways because it's enjoyable and almost obligatory to the community. The farmer's market is just something that should be done.

I've been on both sides of the farmer's market. At first I was the buyer. I came for a week's worth of greens, fruit, eggs, high quality meat, honey, and to get in on the seasonal items before they were gone. The food was good, but I was also interested in talking to the growers and hearing a little bit about the food. It gave me a portal to peer into organic farms and led to my first volunteer day. Fast forward a couple years and I found myself working the farmer's market myself. I was coming to make sales, but most importantly I wanted people to eat the good food and experience the good feeling. I wanted buyers to see how fresh the food was so they could understand the difference between organic and conventional.

The reality of farmer's markets in the back end is sometimes unromantic. Fake farmers who flip bulk Costco extras dominate on low prices. Most of the tents are hot food and the few food growers get passed by. There's no grass or seating, only concrete, so people don't linger. It rains, and no one shows up. You leave after so many hours of work- harvesting, processing, setting up, working the booth, and breaking down with only a couple hundred bucks and wonder why you still do it. But you might meet one future farmer who really, really cares, and that makes all the difference.

For most farmers, even small-time growers, farmer's markets are more for community and fun than for business purpose. The marketing and networking are nice, but it's more of an excuse to get off the farm and hang out with your neighbor farmers than for the money. Farmer's markets are finnicky in a way that other sales channels aren't.

Once you establish a solid connection with a restaurant you can keep that client as long as you please each other. If you grow decent volume, grocery stores are a much more efficient way to unload. If you care about getting your food directly to the customer, community supported agriculture programs are a way to do it more consistently. But still, we do the farmer's markets.

Once again, farmer's markets are on the rise. The numbers are growing. More people care. More people are attending. They won't replace grocery stores, but they don't have to, because the purpose is different. The farmer's market is not just about getting groceries, it is about celebrating food culture and integrating it deeper into your life. Farmer's markets are the meeting points between grower, seller, buyer, and eater. It's technically not necessary, but without it, something would be missing from The Food Life.

Community Supported Agriculture

Small farms in our communities need our help. It would be nice if they could easily succeed on their own. While there's some indication they have a better chance of surviving than the average small business, they have additional obstacles of variant weather, limited growing season, and competition from government supported large-scale agriculture. There is an invisible tax on most good food when you consider the subsidy the government pays to the biggest producers of corn and beef. The price we pay at McDonalds is artificially lowered by government controls. Fake prices for fake food. The small local farms don't benefit from these subsidies so while sometimes the cost of good food may seem high, it is the true price of real food.

Community Supported Agriculture (CSA) is the idea that we should support our local farms by working directly with them to buy our produce. There are several variations of this concept. We can go directly to the farm instead of the grocery store to pick up our produce from the farmers, or the farm may make a weekly delivery run and drop it off on our doorstep. In exchange we buy a farm share which could be a weekly subscription or an upfront lump sum at the start of the season. The benefit to the consumer includes getting to know and trust your growers as well as enjoying the maximum possible freshness of the product.

By the time food makes it the grocery store, it has typically passed many hands and thousands of miles. The growers send it to aggregators who send it to distributors who send it to the supermarkets. There might be a half dozen links in the chain, and with each exchange of hands the food loses freshness, the farmer gets a smaller proportional share of the food dollar, and more fuel is burned. With a CSA system you can reduce the chain of distribution to the bare minimum- just you and the farmer. The farmer gets to maximize their profit and you can even pay a lower price than the store because all the middlemen were eliminated. And of course, you get the freshest food.

It would be nice if Government Support Agriculture included the wave of small farms. That's not to say there's nothing. There are plenty of USDA and other grants out there available to fledgling farmers trying to get their food operation off the ground. But something like across the board tax breaks for food growers could tip the scales and trigger a sea change. That's the most likely way I see us getting back to growing 50% of our food in backyard gardens. And why not? We can still keep the centralized food system for food security but bolstering our local food systems would do wonders for rejuvenating the health and happiness of our people.

We can't wait for the government to step in and help when there's no indication that food quality is on any politician's radars. This duty has been left for the people. If we have time, we ought to plant a few fruit trees in the backyard, a row of greens, and grow some herbs on the back porch. If not, we can vote with our food dollars and support our community farms by going to the land and buying our CSA shares each season.

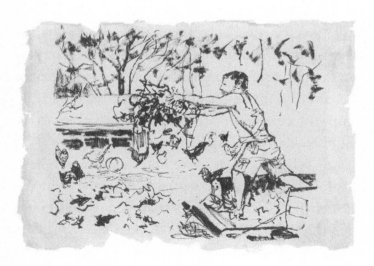

Chickens and Eggs

There's nothing quite like collecting eggs from your own chickens to scramble up for brunch. Especially when you have some leftovers to give to friends, hungry pigs, or sell to the local market for others to enjoy. Thank you to these laying hens for nourishing us with so much nutrition and protein. Crack 'em open, fry 'em up with farm fresh roots, toss in some spice, and enjoy!

Hens are a great lifestyle addition and investment for anyone who wants to get closer to their food. They don't require much space and don't need that much from you. You get a lot back for a little investment. Toss them your extra kitchen scraps, pour them some grain, and watch them pop out tasty eggs for you. Whether you are in the city or the country, it doesn't take much to set up a little coup with cozy nesting roosts for your chickens to lay your breakfast and lunch.

When it comes to feeding chickens, you have to think about the essential chickenness of the chicken. While chickens do enjoy scraps and grain, the chicken expresses its chickenness when it scratches and pecks for bugs. This is ideally how it will get much of its own protein. So when you are farming chickens you also have to think about farming bugs. How can you create an environment where there are more tasty grubs for your chickens to eat? You can start by feeding the bugs, Your chickens might not like leftover citrus fruit, but bugs will, and your chickens will take care of them. Throw down some boards for bugs to live under and flip them over periodically to uncover these tasty treats for your chickens. If you're worried about a runaway bug population, have no fear, the chickens will take care of that.

It's important to keep the environment clean and healthy, and a great way to do that is layering wood chip mulch. This organic matter will create a living bedding that absorbs and breaks down the chicken waste, and keeps the smell down, while also creating an environment for bugs to thrive. The chickens will turn the mulch, scratch and peck for food, and all you have to do is change the bedding every few months.

If you have extra space, your chickens might enjoy roaming pasture and picking bugs from other animal's dung. You could make a portable chicken-mobile on wheels or skis and rotate them behind grazing animals. But don't feel bad if you confine your chickens to a coup though. Historically, unlike grazing animals, chickens have been domesticated more in small stationary houses than pasture, and they are adapted to this. Chickens become hefted to the home. They don't like to roam far because predatory birds or mammals can swoop in on them. They like the familiar protection of the coup. With unclipped wings they can always fly over the fence, but they usually choose not to. Instead, they fly up into their home coup at night for comfortable security. This makes chickens the easiest, most manageable farm animal and source of animal protein you can raise. Give them some love and enjoy their eggs with your friends and family.

Trees of Hope

Imagine if every city sidewalk was lined with fruit trees. Imagine if every ornamental suburban lawn was a food forest. Imagine kids picking fresh ripe fruit after school instead of eating candy and fast food. Why not? I see a lot of excuses. People say it's hard to implement, trees are buggy, and that it's messy. Whose responsibility is it? Whose fruit is it? So the governments say forget it, this is more trouble than it's worth. The people don't know how long they'll be living here, so why bother. Let's stick with the same system we have despite skyrocketing obesity and disease. Me? I say plant a tree.

A tree is a symbol of hope. Planting a tree says, "I want to create a better future, right here in this spot, and I'm willing to wait for it." It takes imagination, patience, and foresight beyond today's problems, even years ahead. It's not hard, expensive, or time consuming. Anyone can start from discarded fruit seeds. A people who say it's not worth it to plant trees have little hope for the future. A people who look around and see no one planting trees have little inspiration to do it themselves. Someone has to step up and be Johnny Appleseed. The hope of one person really can change the landscape.

In the past year we've transplanted over 200 baby fruit trees. We dig holes, irrigate, compost, mulch, weed, prune, and protect. While I have no legal ownership of the land, it connects me to the land in a way that many land owners don't get to experience. I hope to live to see the orchard blooming rich with lemons, limes, oranges, mangos, avocados, papayas, bananas, coconuts, and figs. My tongue salivates just thinking about the future.

Walking out my front door I pass two mango trees. Walking out my backdoor I pass a starfruit tree and a fig tree. When in season, I can pick a piece of fruit on my way to or from work. I didn't plant these trees. Someone planted them decades ago. Someone had to have a vision of the future that is richer, more vibrant, and more nutritious. A few small actions, and fruit for decades. A better future. A better life for the next generation.

Trees deserve respect. These ancient creatures were here long before us, and they will be here long after us. Some can live for hundreds, if not thousands of years. We tend to think of them as still, dull, almost lifeless, but they are smart. They communicate with each other in several ways. Trees produce pheromones to warn neighbors of impending threats. By the time insects arrive a tree may have already bittered and hardened its leaves thanks to an alarm from a friend. Trees link their roots, and with the help of fungus create vast sugar sharing and information networks with the next related tree across the whole forest. Trees support each other better when planted in a triangle rather than a straight line, and baby trees grow better with the support of a nurturing mother. They have social systems beyond our comprehension, a kind of sentience in their connected root brains beyond our understanding.

We think we have domesticated fruit trees, but they may have domesticated us. They tricked Adam and Eve with their tasty fruit to propagate them. Our lives have become intertwined with theirs, and our destinies depend on theirs.

The best thing about our Tree of Hope Orchard is that it has been funded primarily through donations. It's not a hard sell. Anyone who is concerned about the future can see that trees are part of the answer. If they don't have the energy to plant a tree themselves, they are in full support of us planting it for them. There are multiple levels of participation. You can vote with your dollars and your stomach. You can create hope for a generation by planting trees.

Small Growers Unite

At the peak of mango season we have two thousand pounds of mangos coming through our food hub every week. Our wash station becomes a crowded, sticky mess requiring constant sorting of mangos into different stages, trying to get each batch out the door at the right time. While we currently have several dozen mango trees on our property for shaded snack breaks in the summer months, most of the mangos we handle aren't ours- they're brought in by backyard growers from the surrounding valley. Someone in their family planted a mango tree years back, and the ripening fruits hit the valley all at once. It's too much for us all to eat, so someone needs to run a food hub for collecting and distributing the fruit, and that's what we do.

Critics of small-scale organic, biodiverse, regenerative, integrity food systems claim it doesn't scale well. But when you look at the numbers, the truth is it could actually scale better than the concentrated food system. Small scale operations on average produce more food yield per acre. Yes, they require more labor, but they result in fewer sick casualties put out of work. They tend to be more environmentally friendly and much cheaper for delivery because they can spread out and cluster around city centers instead of concentrating far from the population. But if we do need more land, we have it. There are 40 million acres of ornamental lawns in the USA that could be repurposed for gardens and orchards. The problem isn't that it can't scale, it's how complex the scaling is. It's easier to scale a 10,000-acre mono crop operation with robotic tractors, pesticides, herbicides, and irrigation than 10,000 one-acre organic plots, but that doesn't mean it can't be done, and it doesn't mean we can't grow more food that way either.

Part of the solution of solving scaling issues is regional food hubs- buyers for backyard growers who collect, sort, and ready produce for distribution. Another important tool is distribution systems between the farm hubs and the end buyers- support for marketing, transactions, and distribution. We don't do that, but we work with companies who do and they are helpful to us. Not every grower needs to know every business skill. They should be focused on growing the best food they can. Let other people do the processing and delivering. It's complicated, it involves a lot of moving parts, but it works, and it builds a picture of how local food systems can feed way more people better food.

The world doesn't yet need food hubs in every region. In many places there just aren't enough small time growers or backyard fruit trees. This is an existing solution for a future question of what we will do when more individuals start growing food right where they are. Let the people grow food, and we will make it work.

During mango season, the food hub becomes our main business, even outproducing the food that we grow ourselves. This isn't by choice. It's by need of the community. But as the season winds down, our work continues as growers bring in avocados, coconuts, cucumbers, dragon fruit, papayas, bananas, citrus, soursop, jackfruit, and various other tasty fruits. We snack on them, we feed the extras to our animals, and we flip 'em for people and profit. Through our combined efforts we do the best we can to take the abundance of fruit growing in our region and feed the whole island.

The Future is Food

Looking at the future of food, I see two divergent possibilities. The first is extremification of the modern mass food system- more animals in less space, more heavily processed food, bigger mono crops on fewer farms, more laboratory farming, vertical farming, giant concentrated bug farming operations, more food, but more sick, dysfunctional people and societies. The second is a return to The Food Life. More young labor fleeing modern life, their white collar jobs replaced by robots, returning to the land, growing diverse crops for nutrition and taste. My bet is both happen at the same time.

Extremification of concentrated food production and mass distribution is a given. All the momentum pushes this way. We have billions more people coming, and we must feed them. Nothing else scales as big and easily. Technology and artificial intelligence will allow fewer and fewer people to grow more and more food. Robots will figure out better ways to feed all these mouths. There's no way around it.

Yet I'm optimistic small-scale intensive agriculture will boom as a secondary supporting system that helps feed healthier people and society. To feed all these extra people we need higher yields from our land, and biodiverse organic farming is the way to do it. It's proven to be more productive per acre, with the downside being the inefficiency of requiring intensive human labor. But as technology and AI take off, billions of people will be freed from all areas of work and need something productive to do. I see many of these people growing food, because it's needed, it's wanted, and the conditions will allow it.

An ideal system probably has both centralized and local food operations. Centralized food systems prevent localized famines; localized food systems prevent widespread famine and disease. We need both to work. The centralized food system has plenty of help, but localized food can always use more energy. It's for the good of humanity, and it also makes for great lives, and good food too. It's hard to predict the future of food, but easy to predict that more people will want and choose The Food Life. Will you?

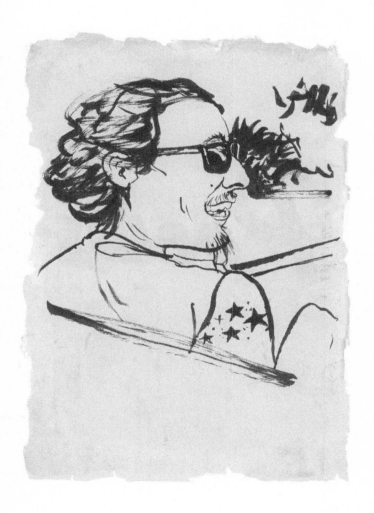

Poems

Sun warmed cheeks
Rain kissed brows
Wind breath on the hair
Birdsong on the ears
The grass dances green
A rooster crows
The sheep bleat
A pig oinks
Soft soil beneath our feet
Hugged by gravity
Held by the Earth
We sow our seeds

Wind and sun in my face
Sheep at my back
Headed for greener pastures
Flashback to childhood- a sheepskin blanket
Flashback to past lives- ten thousand years herding
sheep on the plains
I feel the shepherds blood in my veins
The sheep dance and chew around me
Green grass and leaves in bunches
Face down, ass up
Down she goes!
I love my sisters, mothers, brothers, sons
One bad ass dad
They weed the orchard
Manure into the soil
Back to the Earth
Thank you my friends

Life can be so so so good
Vivid colors
Beautiful people in
Beautiful scenes
Clouds bursting over mountains
Hot sunsets over blue waters
Birds, bees, breeze, and trees
Good food clean air
Soily feet and sandy hair
Sun on the skin
Good missions
Good teams
Hard work that matters
Rustling leaves and
Sweet harmonies
Community that cares

Holy shit look at those mountains
They're popping off the face
Oh my God blue skies and clouds so bright
The green grass dances around me, the trees smile
I feel the kiss of the wind, the love of the sun
The soil beneath my feet is simply incredible
My body is warm and buzzing
So much love and joy to be outside in nature
I think the mushrooms are kicking in

Good

Reads

"Guns, Germs, and Steel" by Jared Diamond
"Sapiens: A Brief History of Humankind" by Yuval Noah Harari
"The Food Explorer: The True Adventures of the Globe-Trotting Botanist Who Transformed What America Eats" by Daniel Stone
"Letters to Young Farmers: On Food, Farming, and Our Future" by Stone Barns Center
"The Good Life" by Helen and Scott Nearing
"The Shepherd's Life" by James Rebanks
"The Dirty Life: A Memoir of Farming, Food, and Love" by Kristin Kimball
"Animal, Vegetable, Miracle: A Year of Food Life" by Barbara Kingslover
"The Sheer Ecstasy of Being a Lunatic Farmer" by Joel Salatin
"Folks, This Ain't Normal: A Farmer's Advice for Happier Hens, Healthier People, and a Better World" by Joel Salatin
"You Can Farm: The Entrepreneur's Guide to Start and Succeed in a Farming Enterprise" by Joel Salatin
"The Omnivore's Dilemma" by Michael Pollan
"Holy Shit: Managing Manure to Save Mankind" by Gene Logsdon

"The Vegetarian Myth: Food, Justice, and Sustainability" by Lierre Keith
"Food and Power in Hawaii: Visions of Food Democracy" by Kimura and Suryanata
"The Blue Zones: 9 Lessons for Living Longer from the People Who've Lived the Longest" by Dan Buettner
"Pottenger's Prophecy" by Graham, Kwesten, and Scherwitz
"The Hidden Life of Trees: What They Feel, How they Communicate- Discoveries from a Secret World" by Peter Wohlleben
"The Inner Life of Animals: Love, Grief, and Compassion- Surprising Observations of a Hidden World" by Peter Wohlleben
"The Secret Life of Plants: a Fascinating Account of the Physical, Emotional, and Spiritual Relations Between Plants and Man" by Peter Tompkins
"The Farm on the Roof: What Brooklyn Grange Taught Us About Entrepreneurship, Community, and Growing a Sustainable Business" by Anstasia Cole Plakias
"It Takes Cow Chips to Make Dinner: Growing Up in Rural South Dakota in the 30's and 40's" by L. Dale Redlin

Made in the USA
Coppell, TX
23 January 2021

48667830R20125